No Regrets

Advance Praise

You will find Rayna Neises book, *No Regrets, Hope for Your Caregiving Season*, a book that you will return to time and time again. You will want to absorb the remarkable wisdom she shares along the entire journey of caring for your loved one. With her wit, wisdom, knowledge, and first-hand experiences, you will find both help for you as well as care for your parent. In spite of the challenges, her main themes of hope and joy for them and for you permeate her writing. *"Finding ways to bring your parents joy will keep them happier and with you longer.....thinking about the things you already know about them and then figuring out how you can adapt those things to allow them to continue to engage as long as possible."* After all, isn't it all about loving them with no regrets? You will be so glad you have this book on your shelf and Rayna whispering in your ear.

—**Nancy Booth**, Author, Spiritual Director

Rayna Neises delivers on her promise to provide hope for your caregiving season in her book, *No Regrets*. Told from a powerful first-person perspective, readers will happily (even gratefully) discover hope, encouragement, as well as a treasure trove of practical suggestions for journeying through the caregiving season. Neises knows from first-hand experience both the triumphs and the tragedies of giving care to loved ones, and she passes on her wisdom and knowledge in a winsome, uplifting way. Highly recommended.

— **Michele Howe**, author of 25 books for women and families. Her newest release is *Giving Thanks for a Perfectly Imperfect Life.*

Every page of Rayna Neises' book is filled with wisdom, compassion and profound insights. Reading it is like walking alongside your best friend, only this best friend has embarked on the journey before and is now along to support, instruct, encourage, and motivate you. Her intentional approach to caregiving will broaden and deepen your own experience, enabling you to also discover the joy and satisfaction in caring for another. In *No Regrets*, Rayna shares the beautiful heartfelt story of caring for her parents, and her passion to assist other caregivers.

—**Kelly Johnson**, Co-founder of Nourish for Caregivers; Co-author of *The Caregiver's Companion*

I have never thought I could take care of my mom, if she should need me to, before she dies. But after reading Rayna's book, she inspired me to at least try so I would have no regrets when my mom is gone. Besides all the tips she gives on caregiving for a loved one, the second part of the book is full of ideas for caring for ourselves, too. Be sure to grab a tissue as you read about the trials and struggles Rayna went through in caring for her Dad.

—**Sharon Witzell**, Program Coordinator Senior Adult Ministries Catholic Diocese of Wichita

The perfect blend of insight, understanding, and practical guidance, Rayna Neises brings hope and wisdom to anyone caring for a parent. *No Regrets* is so incredibly valuable because it focuses on what matters most to every caregiver...the ability to look back on the journey you've walked as a caregiver to your parent and being able to say you have no regrets. Yes, there will be heartaches. By reading this book and learning from its rich stories, you will begin to exchange your heartaches for hope and memories to forever cherish.

—**Debra Kelsey-Davis**, Co-author of *The Caregiver's Companion*; Co-founder of Nourish for Caregivers

I strongly recommend *No Regrets* for anyone who is a caregiver or who desires to support caregivers. This book shares heartwarming caregiver experiences and practical steps at the same time. I love the easy to read layout of the book. I'm a caregiver, and I understand what it takes to care for a parent at home. If I had access to this book at the beginning of my journey, it would have saved me time, money, and heartache. This is a must-have book, because there is a high likelihood that most of us will either need a caregiver or be a caregiver before our life journey ends.

—**Karen Weaver**, Springdale, MD

In this personal journey as a caregiver, Rayna shares her reliance on deep and abiding faith through all of the emotions she experienced, the ability to embrace the good moments and balance the tough ones, and the impact of caregiving a family member on her other relationships. Of great value to the reader, she shares what she learned and how others might process their own unique experiences through the lens of her wisdom. The takeaway we can gain from Rayna is knowing when to trust oneself, when to trust the family collective and when to trust outside expert sources.

—**Laura Beth DeHority**, Licensed Marriage and Family Therapist, San Jose, CA

Rayna's ability to share in words her journey of caregiving is like hearing the stories in person as they were occurring. You feel the emotion, the heartache, and indescribable and unconditional love she has the capacity to give as a daughter, a sister, a wife, and caregiver.

—**Stephanie Gaskill Jakub**, Realtor & Designer

As Rayna's pastor I had a front row seat to the story that inspired this book. I watched with both admiration and helplessness. I admired her determined care for her father. Yet I felt helpless to provide guidance in this situation that went beyond my own experience and knowledge. I remember wishing I had a resource to assist her and me. Now I have that resource in her book *No Regrets: Hope for Your Caregiving Season.*

This is the book I've needed for many years and a resource I will share widely with people under my care. Rayna combines her own experience, the wisdom of others, and the message of Jesus Christ to tell the weary caregiver, "There is always hope." That's the message I want to put in the hands of those I counsel.

Rayna writes early on, "Caring is not a one-size-fits-all situation." What follows is not a step-by-step plan. Rather, Rayna addresses the many worlds that comprise the caregiver's universe and provides wisdom that empowers action. This is a book that cares for caregivers and will be an invaluable tool for my pastoral ministry.

—**Cody Busby**, Senior Pastor

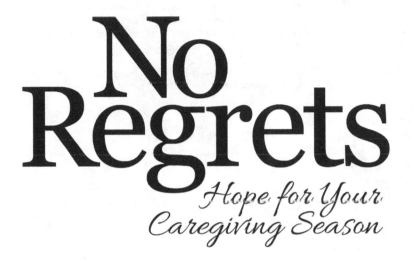

No Regrets

Hope for Your Caregiving Season

RAYNA NEISES

NEW YORK

LONDON • NASHVILLE • MELBOURNE • VANCOUVER

No Regrets

Hope for Your Caregiving Season

© 2021 Rayna Neises

Published in New York, New York, by Morgan James Publishing. Morgan James is a trademark of Morgan James, LLC. www.MorganJamesPublishing.com

ISBN 9781631953446 paperback
ISBN 9781631953453 eBook
Library of Congress Control Number: 2020946924

Cover Design by:
Rachel Lopez
www.r2cdesign.com

Interior Design by:
Christopher Kirk
www.GFSstudio.com

Unless otherwise noted, scripture is taken from the Holy Bible, New International Version®, NIV® copyright ©1973, 1978, 1984, 2011 by Biblica, Inc.® Used by permission. All rights reserved worldwide.

Scripture marked KJV is taken from the King James Version of the Bible, public domain.

Scripture marked NLT is taken from the Holy Bible, New Living Translation, copyright © 1996, 2004, 2015 by Tyndale House Foundation. Used by permission of Tyndale House Publishers Inc., Carol Stream, Illinois 60188. All rights reserved.

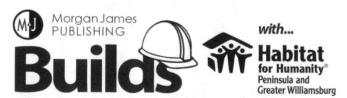

Morgan James is a proud partner of Habitat for Humanity Peninsula and Greater Williamsburg. Partners in building since 2006.

Get involved today! Visit
MorganJamesPublishing.com/giving-back

For my first loves.

My daddy ~ Thank you for teaching me what living out love looks like, for being the best coach, business partner, and Dad ever and for always having faith in me.

My mom ~ Thank you for being my biggest cheerleader in all the things, the wisdom and compassion you shared and the love that was easily seen every day in our home growing up.

To my forever love, my Farmer. Thank you for being a man of deep faith and integrity, bringing me "home" to the farm and supporting me in living out love for my dad. Your love and confidence in me make me a better person.

For my sister, Robin. Thank you for being my sister by birth, my friend by choice, and my right hand throughout this season. In some ways, we couldn't be more different, but we're the same in all the important ways.

Table of Contents

Acknowledgments

Writing this book was a labor of love. I would never claim to be a writer, so I laughed it off when Paula Jones, the director of the day stay program my dad attended, told us at his funeral that we needed to write a book. But when other colleagues, friends, and family also commented about how our experience would be of great benefit to families/adult children who find themselves in a caring season, I finally listened. It took many amazing people to create this book of hope.

First and foremost, I have to say I am the person I am today only because of the love and sacrifice of my Lord, Jesus Christ. His example of selflessness while living on this earth has been a model I have sought to emulate throughout my life. I am eternally grateful that He blessed me with parents who also lived a life of integrity and love.

My Farmer, a man of hard work and few words. Thank you for giving me permission to figure out what was best for Dad and supporting us every step of the way. Your willingness to share me with my dad and family, give of yourself, and always provide a strong shoulder to lean on will never be forgotten.

The amazing team of caregivers who learned to love me, my family, and my dad made it all possible. There were so many of them over the four-and half-year period; I cannot name them all. I am so grateful. To the staff at Shalom Day Stay Program, we are so sad to hear you are no longer able to serve families like ours. You had a significant and positive impact on our journey.

Dr. Rowden, your understanding, expertise, and compassion forever impacted us and our ability to do all that we could for Dad in his final years. Without you, our journey would have been much more difficult. Thank you!

Johanna, Sylvia, Martha, Mary, Brian, and Al, your dedication was a blessing. Thank you, Lois, who walked with us from the very beginning to the last days. And Sarah, who helped us walk Dad all the way home. I'm not sure what we would have done without your presence and support.

My sister, Robin Crick, and her eye for details and organization kept us all going strong. John, Delaney, and Jeremey, thank you for the way you loved and supported both Grandpa and your wife/mom during this important season of our lives. He loved you all more than you can know.

Aunt Colleen, the encouragement and support you showed us each step of the way served as a guiding light in the journey. I know doing life without Dad has been hard, but we are thankful to still share it with you.

Nancy Booth, your prayers, insight, and encouragement throughout my caring season were more important than you realize. Your passion for the Lord and for writing has made this book possible in so many ways.

Chris and Jim Howard, thank you for believing in my message and making it possible to create this book. Without your support and vision, I would not have gotten to this point. Thank you to your editing team at vocem, LLC, led by Cortney Donelson, for doing all the hard work of following the rules, which allowed me to share my heart and not worry about it.

Morgan James Publishing, thank you for getting behind this message and making it possible for me to share our story and the hope that intentionally caring for your loved ones brings. To Gayle West, my author relations manager, and the entire Morgan James team, it was a blessing to have your guidance on a book I am so proud to have my name on.

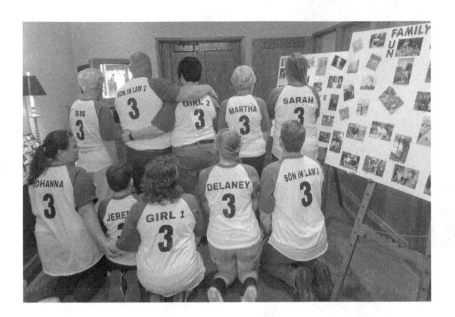

Foreword

Here is what I've learned from losing a parent and from the countless stories I've heard from friends and loved ones—it's not going to look like you think it will.

It was 2014 and life was going pretty much as planned. I was writing books, raising my family, loving my husband, and doing life. Then one day when I called my mom, I could hear the exhaustion in her voice growing deeper and deeper.

My dad was not in great health, but that was nothing new. As a reformed smoker and a daily consumer of a six pack of Coke and a bag a day Cheeto habit, healthy routines had never been one of his hallmarks. But now, the problems were escalating, and he wasn't recovering like he used to. Not only was it taking a toll on my dad, it was starting to affect my mom deeply. And that's when our family had to start making plans for how we were going to navigate this new phase of life.

Rayna can relate—in Chapter 6 she shares, "The changes were right there on my doorstep, and I was not expecting this at all." Trips were cancelled and schedules made. Later, hospice was called, and experts were brought in to help us navigate Dad living and dying at home. In addition, we had to support Mom and each other, because, while Dad was dying, the rest of us had to figure out how to keep on living. Rayna's advice on compromise in this caregiving season would have been so helpful to have.

At the time, I was doing research into how to navigate all these changes, support not only my mom but also my kids, and continue bringing in an income to make all of this possible. The resources available to us as a family were slim, dry, and in some cases, very guilt-producing.

No Regrets, Hope for Your Caregiving Season validates that caregiving can be a very lonely place. I know this from experience. We traveled this journey with very little outside help. While Rayna's book is one to be read from cover to cover, it's also one that can be used over and over as reference for so many aspects of walking your loved one home.

I'm grateful that, in these few short years since my father passed away, at home, surrounded by people he loved and who loved him, Rayna is giving a new, more empowering and powerful way to discuss how to love someone—and each other—well during the hardest time of life. And I'm grateful to Rayna for being a strong hand on our arm, not only guiding us through but also holding us up as we love and let go.

Kathi Lipp
Author, Keynote Speaker, Podcaster

Dear Loving Daughter/Son,

Your heart for your parent's health and happiness is fragile. This season will be filled with heartbreak and blessing!

There will be more questions than answers, more required conversations than you can imagine, and more memories to be made in this season than you can fathom. You will grow tired, but don't give up! It will be worth it.

I know you can walk your parent all the way home while preserving a life that you love, one with no regrets.

Rayna

Introduction

O n June 29, 2018, I buried my dad with NO REGRETS!
I realize that not everyone can say that after losing a
parent, but I hope that you will. My prayer is that you have
picked up this book early, before you are very far along in your caring
season for your aging parent. But no matter when you read it, I know
you will find things you can be intentional about so that you, too, can
say you have no regrets.

As a certified life coach, I have walked alongside others through
different life transitions. Sometimes, what you do for others can be
hard to do for yourself. I learned this during my latest caring season,
supporting my dad during his fourteen-year journey with Alzheimer's
disease. Our family decided to honor his wishes by helping him stay
at home throughout his journey by providing the support he needed.

In the beginning, it was more emotional support, but as his disease
progressed, his needs grew and he required more hands-on support.
My sister Robin, my Aunt Colleen, and I were committed to helping
each step of the way. Finally, his independence diminished, and the
three of us, along with a team of paid caregivers, provided twenty-

four-hour care during his final four and a half years when he could not take care of himself.

Through walking this season of caring—negotiating relationships with family members, taking care of my dad, and giving him the best that we could in those last years of his life—I learned more about myself, my family, and the medical field than I ever imagined I would. Once Dad was gone and I walked out of that season, I felt called to step back into caregiving by supporting others who are going through their own journey because it can be a very lonely place to be.

It's difficult to watch your parents age, but it's also a time that can be very rewarding as you help them be as happy and healthy as possible, all the way to the end of their lives.

I'm going to dive into some deep conversations with you about my season of caring in the hopes that it will help you in yours. The choice to keep my father in his home wasn't a hard one, but it was challenging to walk it out all the way to the end. Every decision has a consequence, which is why I want to share this with you. Sometimes, you can see that time is coming, that time when you need to step in and help take care of your parents, but there are also times it can happen quickly, surprising you when you least expect it.

As this book unfolds, I'm going to walk you through some of those challenges and ideas that are imperative for you to know, no matter where you are in this journey. Whether you are planning for when this time comes, if you are just finding out that it's time to start making some decisions, or you are in the thick of this season already, this book will be an invaluable resource for you.

My goal is to help. If you are reading this in the early stages of this journey, able to make decisions before you're in the middle of it, you will make better decisions. When you are under pressure, the brain is wired to stop thinking and only focus on your survival. Being able to pre-determine your choices and be in agreement with your parents about what they really want can make a world of difference. If you've missed that boat, you will still want to bury them with no regrets. Developing the ability to stop in the midst of it, cease reacting, start thinking, and decide what it looks like for you and your family is crucial.

No Regrets is a personal journey of my season of caring and one that I share with you so you can walk your parents all the way home with love and compassion while still having a life to walk back into.

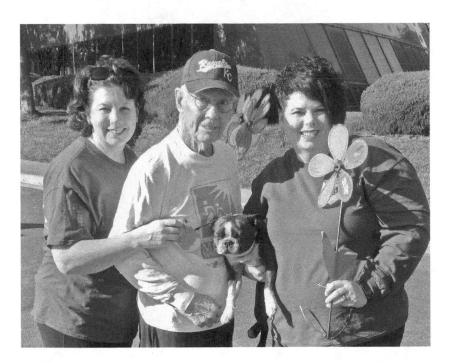

PART 1

Caring for Others

Dear Overwhelmed Daughter/Son,

There are so many things to take care of; no wonder you feel overwhelmed.

You can ask for help. You need to support your parents in their journey home.

Your love for your parent is what everyone sees in all that you do to support them.

Take it a day at a time, and always remember . . . you are an irreplaceable part of their lives.

Rayna

CHAPTER 1

Decisions

Once the decision to keep my father home was made, there was still so much to think about. My sister and aunt were on board to give him a comfortable situation, share our love for him, and allow Dad to live out the remainder of his life in his environment. When you start looking at it and planning for it, there are a lot of options and things to consider before that decision can be made.

Not long after my dad's diagnosis at age seventy-two, we sat down and had a family meeting. We had lost my mom to Alzheimer's just seven years before my dad was diagnosed. We had already been through this journey. My mom had walked through Alzheimer's for twelve years at home with my dad as her primary caregiver. Dad had a little support; he allowed people to come in and help during the day, but overall, he carried the load all the way through Mom's illness. So he knew what he was asking when the one thing he asked of my sister and me was for him to stay at home as long as possible. "As long as possible" was a little vague for me personally.

What does caring for him at home look like,
and how are we going to do that?

We didn't know the answers when he asked for that, but we assured him we would do what we could. That commitment, for me, was a driving force throughout the entire season. How long is as long as possible? For me, it meant as long as I could help Dad be as healthy and as happy as he could be. Those were always my goals—for him to be as healthy and happy as he could be at that stage in his life.

We knew things were going to get worse. We knew that his ability to take care of himself was going to diminish. That is the disease . . . that is Alzheimer's. We weren't sticking our heads in the sand, but we were definitely aware of his desire to be at home. That gave us marching orders to stay true to that commitment.

At the time of my dad's diagnosis with Alzheimer's disease, he was living in his home with his sister. Aunt Colleen is just twenty-five months younger than him; they were always two peas in a pod. About seven years after his Alzheimer's diagnosis, he was diagnosed with melanoma. He had surgery to have it removed, which went very well until he contracted a MRSA infection. MRSA is very nasty, so he had quite a long, confusing, and exhausting stay in the hospital. Combine the infection with the Alzheimer's and the fact that anesthesia can significantly impact brain function, and it was no surprise when Dad's cognitive function went downhill quickly at that point.

He went from functioning at home with his sister on his own, helping with cooking and cleaning, and showering and shaving daily to experiencing a lot of confusion and difficulty taking care of his basic daily needs. My aunt became overwhelmed with being the one person who was caring for him. Even though we brought help in for her, it just wasn't working well. It got to the point where she needed to leave my dad's home for a place of her own. That brought our family to a point where we had to look at our options. Like with most families, the first and seemingly most logical choice was a memory care unit.

Exploring Options

I'll never forget the day I walked out of the memory care unit. I heard that door slam behind me and the lock click in place. As my aunt and I walked down the hall, tears streamed down my face. I thought, "I can't see him there."

My aunt saw my tears and asked, "Honey, what's wrong?"

I said, "I just can't see Dad living there."

My aunt replied, "I know, babe. I can't either." With that simple statement, she quietly went on to her car.

When I got back to my father's house, I was still sad. My husband asked me what was going on, and I explained that I just couldn't imagine my dad being left in that memory care unit. He said, "Then, don't do that. If you need to move here and live with your dad to take care of him, then you need to do that."

It was the first time I felt I had permission to think outside the box. I am so thankful for my husband's wisdom in that situation, giving me the option of finding a different solution. Immediately, I started thinking about what I could make work. Since I lived on a farm two hundred and twenty miles from my dad's house, it was going to be quite a commitment, but with my husband's support, I knew I could figure out something to keep my dad in his home. My sister, aunt, and I had already met with the Alzheimer's Association and had received some information about different resources in the community. I hit the ground running by making phone calls and looking through possibilities, trying to see what was available. From there, I came up with a plan of me living part-time with my dad, part-time with my husband on the farm, and bringing in help to cover the rest of the time.

I started to plan without asking anybody else to be a part of the solution.

As I came up with that plan of living half with dad and half at my home, I took it to my sister and asked her what she thought about it.

I wanted to know if she would be willing to let me do this rather than place him in a memory care unit. That opened the conversation for us to explore what it could look like to keep Dad at home.

This was an important first step. When I went to Robin, I had a plan of how this could be possible and asked if she could be open-minded to doing something different and creative to keep our dad out of the memory care unit. It was important to look at all the options that were available and really put in the forefront of my mind what was best for Dad.

No matter what kind of illness your parent is facing, there are countless resources available. Great organizations are in almost every community to deal with different types of medical issues. Our experience was Alzheimer's and memory care, but there are a lot of opportunities for different kinds of care.

Help can come from many places. Family and friends will be the first people you turn to because they can offer a special level of personal support and caring that someone on the outside can't. There is nothing wrong with asking others for help, too. Don't assume you know the answer they are going to give you, but express understanding if they are unable to help. Thank them for considering it. You don't want to burn that bridge, and perhaps that person may be available to help you in the future. Instead of becoming bitter, stay focused on your goal of getting help for you and your loved one.

There are day-stay options. A lot of people are not aware of that, but many communities have options for adult day care centers. Each center will offer various services, along with a wide array of activities that could vary from exercise to outings and music to games. These centers might also offer meal options to give primary caregivers a respite from the daily routine. They offer you the flexibility of being the primary caregiver but still allow you to integrate what you are trying to do for your parent with your personal life. They may even provide transportation, so this is something that you will want to look at when considering keeping a parent home as long as possible.

Dad loved the day-stay center he attended. We started with just a few days a week and increased the frequency when he was not able to continue some of his other activities. He was able to keep up with a variety of activities at the center, as well as see people he loved and enjoyed being around. The day-stay was a part of his weekly routine for the full four and a half years that we cared from him at home before his passing. It was as much a good option for my sister and me as it was for him.

Between initiating in-home care, family members' help, and the day-stay option, we had as many as thirteen people on our team helping us care for my dad twenty-four seven. Permitting myself to do something different than what everybody else assumed would happen was the very first step in this process. From there, it meant finding and evaluating the available resources to make this thought a reality.

Research, Research, Research

When we first reached the point when we knew we had to make some changes, we went to the Alzheimer's Association as a family. We sat down with a counselor and talked through Dad's needs, the kind of available care options, and the different facilities in the area with dementia care.

Honestly, I didn't particularly think this was a helpful meeting because they were not encouraging us to consider keeping him at home. What my sister, aunt, and I did take away from that meeting was the opportunity to really think and talk it through. This meeting allowed us to hear what the disadvantages and advantages were for our family. It forced us to have the serious conversation about how committed we were to finding the best option for my dad, as a family unit.

So while I didn't think it was a great meeting, we were able to use their resources to make phone calls and find out about the services available in our area. It is important to start with some of those outside resources. It's also important to have conversations with people since there is always something to learn. You'd be surprised what others have been through when you just start talking. Finding out who people know and what organizations they've worked with or what companies they've had experience with can be really helpful.

Whenever possible, it's important not to rush decisions. Our knee-jerk reaction would have been just to place him in that memory care unit like everybody was telling us to do. I think you have to take the time to talk about it as a family, pray over it, think on it, and get everyone on board. We knew my husband was on board. My sister, obviously, had to talk to her husband. She had two elementary-aged kids at the time; we knew the entire family was going to be impacted in order for us to have Grandpa at home. My sister was living within a couple of miles of his house, so if a caregiver didn't show up, if Dad fell, or when he needed to go to the doctor, that was going to fall on her shoulders, so it was imperative we were all a part of that decision.

As we started interviewing in-home care companies to come into the house and care for my dad, we had some really specific things we were looking for. The goal of caring for your parent is making sure they get the care they need.

One of the driving forces for choosing care is understanding who they were as a person, who they are in this new season, and what choices they would make for themselves.

My dad was an accountant. I tell you that to help explain that he was a very routine guy. It cracks me up when I think about it, but he took a bologna and cheese sandwich with an apple and Fritos in a brown bag every day to work for lunch as long as I can remember. Literally, every single day, he ate the same lunch. Some people might think that's disgusting and wonder how anyone could eat the exact same lunch for his whole adult life, but that's what my dad did when he could make the choice. He regimented things. Now, we scheduled everything from breakfast to lunch and all his activities. As a family, it was important for us to have people around us who would respect that system—his system—and keep to the schedules we set.

It wasn't about how the caregiver wanted to accomplish her job. Instead, it needed to be about how my dad would have done it if he could do it himself. We needed his caregivers to know they were there to help him do anything as much as he could, the way he would want to, such as getting out of bed himself, taking a shower every day, shaving every day, applying his deodorant, and brushing his teeth daily. He had a specific order and routine to everything he did.

Alzheimer's affects different parts of the brain. If you can keep the brain active in certain areas, then you can keep those long-term memories longer. That's what we did. Up until he had a blood clot that caused the decline that eventually led to his death, he was still able to do some of those daily tasks. It varied from day to day, but because we had the same routine and offered him the ability to do it himself every day and only assisted him if he couldn't, those routines stayed in place.

Structure Helps

We had a checklist for each caregiver explaining what to do at certain times and on certain days. We were clear about what he would eat and how he liked things to be done. There were some challenges with the companies we worked with because we were so specific in what we were looking for. Not everybody was okay with that. When they weren't, that meant they didn't need to work for us. One of the difficult aspects about handling employment like this was that I'd sometimes have to remind my sister, "You know, we're the ones paying them. They work for us. They need to do what we're asking them to do. If they don't want to, we need to find someone who will."

We had some great caregivers from each company we worked with, but it seemed like the ability for some caregivers to stay committed to our family and our wishes waned the longer we employed them. We required all caregivers who came to care for my dad to be trained by us, so dad would see consistent faces—the same people. We wanted them to have a connection and a relationship with my dad. We would always require each caregiver to come in and meet Dad and us and go through the routine. Then we would monitor how they were getting along with him. It surprised me how often they felt that was just too much to ask.

It was important to me that my dad, my sister, and I got along with the caregivers. We wanted to feel like they were focused on Dad and his best interests throughout the process. If we found that someone's commitment to us was waning, then we would ask for someone else.

It was funny because there were caregivers that my dad connected with that weren't my favorite people. It was fun to see how much he loved them and how different dispositions brought different emotions in him. Each of those relationships was amazing to watch as it developed. I loved supporting and helping him experience that happy, healthy life that I wanted him to have.

It all comes down to what's best for your loved one — the best environment and situations you can provide — and how to make those things happen.

You have to keep these questions at the forefront of your mind so everything you add, every company you work with, every care unit you bring in, and every person you introduce to the scenario, aligns with that mission. If they don't, figure out how to find someone else so that you keep that environment safe for your loved one.

Notes

_____

_____

_____

_____

_____

_____

_____

_____

_____

_____

_____

_____

_____

_____

_____

_____

Dear Bewildered Daughter/Son,

Choices are around every corner. Learn as much as you can about every option. Don't get boxed in and miss some options that might fall outside the box.

Get clear on what is most important to you and your parent. Always keep the big picture in mind, and take the small steps needed to get there. Things become clearer when you keep moving toward what's most important.

The choices are clearer, one choice at a time.

Rayna

CHAPTER 2

Adjust Your Thinking

There are a lot of things that you're going to have to decide when you get to this point. Getting into the right headspace is important when you've been hit with the news that your life is about to change, and you're going to end up moving in a different direction than what you had planned.

There is a cost involved with every decision we make and understanding that on a daily basis, especially in these caregiving situations, is crucial. Even if it's just choosing to spend money on a vacation, that money can only be spent on the vacation. It can't be spent on your retirement fund or buying a new car.

Deciding to spend half of my week living with my dad versus on the farm with my family came at a price but deciding to put him in a facility would have been at a cost as well. I would have lost my dad without having the cherished memories, the laughter, and the love, which we experienced day in and day out during those four and a half years.

Never forget there is a cost with both choices,
whatever direction you go.

I encourage you to stop and look at it with clear eyes, and get everybody in agreement. My husband and I had a high school student at home at the time I traveled to care for Dad. That meant I missed things. I didn't get to attend all of his Scholar's Bowl Competitions, but I did get to see my nephew play basketball with my dad. I missed my grandson's first birthday party, but I also got to experience my dad's last birthday party. There were only three of us at Dad's final birthday, but it was still a celebration of his day. If I hadn't missed one, I would have missed the other. In this journey, there are tough decisions to be made. While going through it, you must remember to be kind to yourself and realize you are only one person; you can't be in two places at once.

Think Long Term

These days, we live in a very here and now mindset, only thinking in the immediate. It's important to slow down and think about the long term, not just for you but also for your parent. It's keeping the benefits for your parent in mind, putting them in an environment where they can be comfortable and where they can live as normal a life as possible.

As you're stepping into the role of caring for your parent, it's important to remember that they cared for you when you couldn't care for yourself. That's all we're doing for them. As our parents age, their needs increase. All of us come into this world not able to do anything on our own. We need someone to feed us, burp us, and soothe us—we have so many needs! The amount of our needs is significantly high.

As we grow up, we become independent. So much so that we get to the point of not even thinking we need anybody (like most teenagers). Then there is the season of life when we're all adults—our parent is an adult, we have become an adult, and life goes on that way for quite a long while.

The next change that happens in this circle of life is that our parents' needs start to increase. We've never been in this role before. We've never been the one who's been more confident at handling life than our parents. They reach a point where they have more needs than we do, they cannot take care of themselves the way they always have. Oftentimes, you hear people refer to this as "role reversal." You start parenting your parent.

I, personally, don't like that thought process. I don't feel like it's true. If I had talked to my dad as if he were my child or like a toddler, he would have probably acted more like one. He would have thrown a fit and been unwilling to help. Treating him as an adult who simply had needs he couldn't meet for himself allowed me to love him well, honor him, and care for his needs.

This is a season of life where your parent's needs are going to increase and are going to be greater than you've ever seen in your lifetime. The highest level of need will be just before they pass, unless it's an unexpected death. It's a season, one that we need to step into to help meet their needs. I think keeping these truths in mind is helpful. They're not going to be here permanently and their needs are not going to be this high forever.

Don't think of it as parenting your parent.
You are simply meeting needs they can't meet for themselves.

Think big picture. What will you regret when they're no longer here? I think you'll regret the time you didn't get to smile, hug, or simply spend time with them. You don't want to have those regrets when you look back. Having the ability to understand how much you're going to receive in those times of meeting their needs helps you to make the sacrifices that may be required.

That's part of what we were looking for in caregivers, as well. We wanted people who saw Dad as a person with needs to be met, which, in this season, he couldn't meet himself. We know Alzheimer's affects the brain in bizarre ways. People forget who their loved ones are, but a week before my dad passed away, I was standing at the head of his bed where he couldn't see me. Dad asked, "Where's Rayna?" I can't remember the last time I had heard my name come from his lips, but I'll always remember that as the last time I heard him say my name. We don't know exactly what they know and what they don't, if they really are there and just can't communicate it or not.

What I do know is my dad had joy in me being with him. Whether he knew I was his daughter or not, he knew that he loved me. That love was always there. When we had been faced with the process of losing my mom years earlier, one thing I noticed was when I talked to her before I came in the room, her face would light up. She recognized my voice. My body didn't match what her brain thought I should look like, but she knew who I was in her own way. There is more going on inside people with Alzheimer's than we realize I think—way more than they can communicate with us.

Whether our parents are mentally impaired or not, they can be very prideful. All of us are. I think it's hard for them to be honest with us, and say, "I miss you. I just want you here." Aging and becoming dependent on those around us is a scary process, no matter who you are. Knowing the people you love the most are right there with you, going through it with you, definitely makes a difference.

Choosing the Right Care

When it comes to how to take care of a parent, I think every family must make decisions for what's best for their particular family. Caring is not a one-size-fits-all situation. For instance, with my mom, it was tougher for her to stay in the home because she didn't negotiate stairs well, and there were stairs in our home. But on the other hand, she was more of a homebody, so she enjoyed staying home and was much less anxious when she was there. My dad was very physically fit and was able to negotiate those stairs all the way until he formed the blood clot and had surgery. He was also very social, so staying at home only was not best for him.

Look at all of the different needs your parent has, and see what's going to work best for your family.

Financial restraints will also dictate some of what's possible. We were able to pay people to come to him and not have to send him to a residential facility. Not everybody has the resources required for in-home care. It's important that you know your parent's wishes but it's just as important that you understand your family's abilities.

As previously mentioned, my sister lived two miles away from my dad's home. If she wasn't that close, I'm not sure our plan would have worked. It might have had to look very different if we didn't have someone close by. The fact that there was a distance of over two hundred miles from my home to Dad's did have an impact on what our decisions had to be. This is where the decision of living part-time with my husband and part-time with Dad came into play.

When I first started traveling to my dad, I was teaching part-time, four days per week. I did that for six months. When I realized caregiving was going to be more of a long-term situation than initially expected, my husband and I made a decision **for** me to resign that teaching position and work from home, so I would be able to contribute to our income but also take care of my dad.

Finances must be considered in this situation—both your parent's ability to pay for the help they need and your ability to be available to step in and offer that help. The one thing many people don't realize is even when your parent is in a home, they still need the support of someone who knows what's going on.

Staying involved, visiting frequently, and understanding what's happening with their health are all very important responsibilities. Yes, the care home will take them to their doctor's appointments, but how much do you know about the medications they're on? How involved are you in what's going on? It'll still take time and energy to invest in your parent as they age.

A parent requiring twenty-four-hour care is definitely challenging. Finding responsible people who are able to be there and who are the right fit for your family can be daunting. It takes a lot of work, no matter which direction you go. Consider the physical care needs of your parent—bathing, feeding, and safety—but there are also core needs, which are being seen and understood.

Knowing you have them in the right place is knowing they're being seen as a person—respected, honored, and cared for.

Near the end of my season of caring, we found ourselves in a place where a decision had to be made once again for my dad. He had that surgery for a blood clot and discharged to a rehabilitation facility for three weeks afterward. At that point, we had to ask ourselves once again, where does he go after he leaves rehab? Can he go home? Does he need a long-term care solution? Once again, we sat down and looked at our options as a family. We decided we could prepare his basement for him to live at the house and avoid stairs. Dad was able to come home.

His heart was aimed at home. There was no doubt about that. After being home for two days, I saw a change in him. It was like he exhaled and relaxed. Even though he was now in the basement, he knew he was at home. Within nine days, he passed away. We weren't expecting that. He was walking; he was eating; he was chattering with us, but then he was done. We were able to feel okay, find a measure of peace with that, because we gave him what he wanted.

Care Needs Versus Core Needs

We can change so much physically around the patient that it ultimately could affect him or her in a negative way. You have to think not only about your parent's care needs but also their core needs, which I briefly mentioned earlier. In order to do that, you need to think about who the person is and who he or she was before this season. Then consider what kinds of things you incorporate to get that sense of normalcy for them.

When I first left that memory care unit that we toured for my dad, I could not see him spending the rest of his life is such a small space. While he couldn't live alone, he was still active at that point. He was playing volleyball three times per week, working out at the gym three days a week, and engaging in life. He loved doing those things. Taking all of those physical activities away from him would have been taking life from my dad.

That was part of the challenge for our family—asking how we could continue to allow him to do what he could do and what he loved to do as long as possible. That was always the goal. Even as we brought in twenty-four-hour care, part of the schedule included taking him to play volleyball and lift weights at the gym three times a week. When I was in town with him, one of our regular activities was going to the gym to lift weights together. Those were the activities he loved to do, and we did them as long as possible.

Maslow's Hierarchy of Needs was something I was taught in school when training to be an educator. Abraham Maslow created a five-tier psychological theory of human needs. The first and most basic of all needs are those to do with physical survival. Then we need to feel safe in the world. Once those needs are met, a need for love, affection, and belonging emerges. From there, self-esteem, or the need to feel of value and to feel respect from others, exists. If the first four needs are being met, a new one will probably develop: the need for self-fulfill-ment, which will eventually get us to a place where we will become the full potential of the person we are created to be.

So it's is important to understand that those basic physical needs have to be met, but full life doesn't exist if only the basic, physical needs are met. When we're too focused on the patient's physical needs, we can miss so many other things. My dad was an accountant. He was a problem solver. We had to keep things in front of him that he could work on and figure out himself in order to support his self-esteem, to keep the essence of who he was as a person.

Having things around you that bring comfort and make your life feel like yours is critical for bringing out your best potential self.

Maslow's Hierarchy of Needs helps us understand how important it is to not just take care of those basic physical needs but to continue meeting the additional core needs, those beyond the basic, survival needs we typically show in caregiving tasks.

Flexibility Counts

It's important during your season of caring to be flexible. Needs today may not be the same needs as time progresses. We may have to adjust how we approach those needs. Flexibility is not one of my strengths, but it's a learned skill. Sometimes, things change temporarily. We went through seasons where Dad had difficulty with his blood pressure, and he was passing out.

Adjusting to needing people who were physically able to pick him up off the floor or needing tools that allowed us to do that, whether it was a hospital bed versus his regular bed, was something we had to do. Within each structure or routine we laid out, we also had to have flexibility within it. Flexibility helps you keep your own sanity when you realize that it doesn't (and won't) have to be exactly the same. It's a matter of doing your due diligence. As you're looking at companies to work with, checking references, and asking people you know who have been in your shoes before what their experiences were are all things you need to do. In the long run, I've learned you really have to go with your gut. If you have concerns, even if you can't name them, it's best just to keep looking. We learned to do a really good job of asking for what we wanted. In the beginning, we were more willing to accept less than that. I would encourage you not to.

*Be very specific with what you want,
and don't accept less than that.*

For us, it was very important to have someone whom Dad knew. His short-term memory wasn't the best, but he interacted with people he was comfortable with differently than he did with strangers. He needed the benefit of the same face waking him up three or four times a week, rather than a new face every day; it made his life better. We were only willing to accept the same two or three people rotating through to take care of Dad. I don't know about you, but I wouldn't want a stranger walking in, waking me up, and telling me to get undressed and into the shower. If a company expected my dad to do that, it wasn't acceptable because that is unrealistic.

Clear Expectations

Communicating clear expectations is important so that everybody on the team knows what to do. When you're talking about care, there can be a lot of gray areas. If you can make things as black and white as possible, then everyone on the team will know what's expected, what's acceptable, and what's not. Having a checklist available so that everyone is on the same page can be very helpful.

While everyone's list will look different, I want to share the evening checklist for my dad. I hope it will help you think about items that should be on your checklist as you navigate your caregiving journey.

CARE TASKS FOR BOB STEEN Updated 10/1/17

PM ROUTINE:

Evening Care Giver	BOB'S BEDROOM/BATHROOM
7:00 PM	Turn down bed covers
	Lay out pj's (drawer or hanging on hook on back of bathroom door)
	Fill and turn on humidifier to lowest setting (far right)
	Get pit White Depends (small black tab deontes back)
	Flush toilet
	Close blinds in bathroom
	Lower both blinds in bedroom
	Tun on lamp on nightstand
	Ensure Bob puts on a White Depends
	Ensure Bob puts on his pj's
	Place Bob's glasses and watch on his dresser w/ mirror
	Place clothes from the day in the laundry basket
	Put shoes in closet
	Set Bed Alarm
	Ensure Bob gets into bed
	Ensure lamp on nightstand is turned out

A requirement for any caregiver has to be that his priority is for the person he's caring for. Anyone who was caring for my dad had to make him the priority. That's why caregivers are there. They are not there to be on their phones or focused on themselves. Their comfort is not my concern. It was about my dad. It was important that Dad liked them and that our family members believed they liked my dad in return. We wanted them to be focused on his care and what was important for him.

I repeatedly said, "Your job is to take care of him and make him as happy as possible, and that means it's about him and doing it his way. Not my way, not your way, and not my sister's way." It's a tough job to be a caregiver, but there are great people out there. You have to keep looking until you find them and let them go when they aren't working out. They may need to find somebody else who is a better fit for them and that is okay.

I had an experience with one caregiver who was not the right person for my dad. Because I lived in the home part-time, even when I was off shift and someone was in taking care of him, I was there. One morning, I was lying in my bed, which was just across the hall from Dad's room, and I heard a caregiver raise her voice and talk down to him. I lay there and listened for a little while; I could tell he was not having a good morning, but the way she was talking to him would have made me angry if I was him. I just couldn't listen to her talk to him that way anymore. I got up, put a robe on, went across the hall, and said, "You're done." She just looked at me. I said, "I need you to leave this room right now. I will take care of getting him ready."

I continued the morning routine with him. He was upset and took more coaxing than usual to get everything done, but I was able to finish getting him ready for the day. The caregiver was in the kitchen when we finished his bedroom routine. She had gotten his breakfast ready to eat. I went on with my morning routine when he seemed fine eating breakfast with her. A short time later, another caregiver came to take Dad to the day-stay facility.

After they left, I asked her what happened, and she said, "I don't know what you're talking about."

"You don't see anything wrong with what happened this morning?"

She replied, "No." We continued to talk, and it was obvious that she really didn't think there was a problem with the way she had spoken to my dad.

I ended the conversation saying, "We don't need you to come back anymore." It seemed simple to me. She had belittled and yelled at my dad. We're all human, and frustration is a part of taking care of someone with Alzheimer's, so I'll be the first to say I yelled at him a few times over the years. The problem was a lack of humility.

Her lack of understanding that what she did wasn't appropriate was what was not okay.

If she yelled at him like that when I was there, I was concerned with what she would do when I wasn't there. Honestly, I was also concerned with what my dad would do. I didn't know if he would put up with being talked to like that for very long. So in this case, that caregiver was not a good fit for us.

My dad loved having male caregivers. They're very hard to find, but there was a gentleman named Al whom Dad just adored. They were like two school-aged kids. It cracked me up to watch them together. Dad would hide behind a door and jump out at Al, and they would laugh. They were such good buddies. Sadly, we lost Al to cancer during the time he was caring for my dad. That was difficult on all of us. The joy that Al brought to his job was greatly missed when he passed.

It was fun to see how the different caregivers brought out different personalities in Dad, and how they enjoyed interacting with him. I would encourage you in this season to find the right people—to find the people who love your loved ones. The group of people that cared for my dad the last two years of his life grieved at his funeral. They had become family. There are people out there who can love like that. That's who you're looking for. Keep searching until you find them.

Options are Available

Oftentimes, we think we're at the mercy of what we are told is available to us. There are lots of options; make sure your loved ones have someone who connects with them. It's important. Make sure caregivers are caring for your loved ones the way they deserve to be cared for. It's empowering to think this way. I've been there and done it. It's not always easy, but you have to do what you have to do. Even as my sister, Robin, and I negotiated through that together, it was an important conversation we had frequently.

If it wasn't working with a caregiver, we learned I was the one to make the phone call. Confrontation or conflict, no matter how professional and respectful, wasn't Robin's strength and she wasn't comfortable having these types of conversations with the companies. Also, I saw more than she saw of the day-to-day interaction the caregivers had with my dad.

The caregivers are providing a service. We are paying them. As long as expectations are made clear at the hiring point, I think you're fair in being able to fire someone for not meeting the outcome you asked for. It goes back to getting in the right headspace, knowing how to think through this. It's not always going to be an easy decision, but now you know at least the option is there, and I hope you can navigate through that better with this advice.

Notes

_____

_____

_____

_____

_____

_____

_____

_____

_____

_____

_____

_____

_____

_____

_____

_____

Dear Special Daughter/Son,

Caring for your parent can bring out the good and the bad in everyone. It is normal to struggle with your loved ones when things are stressful, and you are feeling pulled in many directions.

Don't forget you and your family members have unique gifts and talents to bring to you and your parent's life. You see the big picture and are able to extend grace to everyone.

Your family will always be family, even when your parents are gone.

Rayna

CHAPTER 3

Keeping the Family Intact

I've mentioned my sister, Robin, several times. She and I were a team during this caring season with our dad. Going through times like this can be a big change on the family unit itself. Taking care of a loved one can cause division between siblings and other family members. This will put a whole different pressure on those relationships. My sister and I are extremely different people. I'm not unlike most folks when I say, "I'm not sure how we were raised in the same house by the same parents."

For me, every time I left the driveway at the end of my shift, I said to the Lord, "Okay, I'm tapping out. You're in charge." Not that I thought I was in charge one hundred percent when I was there, but I felt like I was able to do more for Dad there than I was able to do hundreds of miles away. There was a definite division between taking care of Dad and taking care of my family. I had a three-and-a-half-hour drive between those two parts of my life. I had to realize that I had done everything I could do while I was there, and now it was time to put my own family at the center, focus on my work, and do the things that needed to be done at the farm with my immediate family. I had to physically say, "Here he is, Lord. He's yours."

My sister's personality is very different than mine. She never tapped out. She wanted constant contact. When his scheduled time to get up arrived in the morning, she was texting asking if he was awake yet or how he was that day. The minute the caregivers dropped him off at the day-stay facility, she was texting them, asking if he was okay and how the transition went. She needed that interaction with the caregivers even when she wasn't there.

In her caregiving role, my sister's shift was evenings. She went to Dad's house after she put her kids to bed, and she was up early to get her kids ready for school the next day. Dad was asleep when she got there and still asleep when she left, so she didn't see him a lot. During the week, she had one daytime shift on Mondays. Oftentimes, she would schedule his doctor appointments on those shifts. The majority of her job with caregiving was managing the schedule and the other people caring for him, not the hands-on care of my dad. It was very different from my time with him. I couldn't have done what I did with my dad without her. She couldn't have done what she did with my dad without me. We needed each other.

The truth is caregiving brought my family closer.

Robin and I didn't have a very close relationship before this time. There are only two and a half years between us, but our lives were contrasting. I lived out of town. She lived by my parents. She was a professional before she became a mom and then she stayed at home. I was a co-owner of a business and then married a farmer. We lived very different lives. Through this season, we became very close. We knew we needed each other, and we really spent time with each other, supporting one another, checking in on what we could do to help the other through this season.

Communication is Needed

As we were looking at memory care units, I asked her to let me bring him closer to me. She couldn't imagine him being that far away. I knew it mattered to her that he was close. I knew that part of our solution had to be for me to be there with him. When I approached her with the plan to do the caregiving for my dad, I said, "Just let me do this for six months." I tried to plan it all without her being a part of it. But as soon as I showed her the plan, she jumped right on and explained that she could help, she just needed to be sure her kids were in bed by a specific time, and she wanted to be home to get them up and ready for school. When Aunt Colleen saw the plan in the beginning, she said she would like to continue spending time with him, too. She asked if she could take two nights. So we approached it as a team, and that really is the only way this would have worked.

At the end of the first six months, we had another family conversation. We asked each other how it was going? Could we continue this? What do we need to do differently? We made some changes after that discussion. I decided I needed to be home earlier on Sundays to spend time with my husband. Being a farmer, Sunday was the one day he didn't work, so we made some adjustments. I left for Dad's earlier on Thursdays, and I went back home first thing in the morning so we could spend more time together.

As you are trying to build this team with your family, you have to know who they are. You're not going to change them. This situation isn't going to change them. They have the strengths and the weaknesses they have, and they're not you. If you expect them to do and respond and be exactly like you, then you're going to be disappointed, causing tension. Being realistic with the relationships you have and understanding where you're all starting from and who everybody is are important factors to keep in mind. Be realistic.

If there are problems in the relationships now,
they won't magically go away.

You need to use each other's gifts and talents. We learned it was best for me to make the phone calls. When we were looking at interviewing companies to come in and take care of my dad, I did all of that. I gathered the information, laid the groundwork, and communicated the expectations. We decided my sister would be the main contact for them regarding their schedules, so she would meet with them in person or by phone to discuss the details. If we both liked the caregiver company, then we would give it a try. If one of us had a hesitation, we knew we had to keep looking.

It took working with two companies until I learned to say, "This is the way it's going to work. If you hear from me again, your job is in jeopardy. From here on out, you will have all communication with my sister. As long as you keep her happy, you're not going to hear from me. When I make a phone call, something needs to change, or we're going to be looking for another company." As you can imagine, they were oftentimes shocked by that comment but we had to clearly communicate our needs. Eventually, when I had to make that next phone call whenever something wasn't working, I reminded them, "Now remember, I'm giving you this warning. We need this to change, or we're going to be looking for another company."

My sister is so kind-hearted. She would not have been able to be that direct with them. She probably never would have fired anyone. Using our strengths, abilities, and talents to do what we needed to do to care for our dad was definitely the key to us being successful and still loving each other through the process. Giving grace to each other was an absolute must. Let me tell you, we definitely stepped on each other's toes at times. This will happen to you, too.

I recently spoke with Robin about this, and she said, "I think allowing people to do what they want to do, even when it doesn't make any sense to you, is how we made this work." I agreed with her.

Compromise is the key to making everything work.
Everyone gives a little, including the time it takes
to achieve a complete understanding of others' desires.

It made me laugh, because I can think of those things she did, which I thought were crazy. "Why is she doing that?" I thought. Only to find out, she had those same thoughts about some of the things I did, which were important to me. It's critical to have the conversations, even when they aren't easy. We frequently had lunch together on Fridays to check in on life. To be able to enjoy each other and find ways to support each other was important. And you should also have conversations outside of the caregiving roles. Remember, this is a season, and you want to be able to have other things to talk about when this season is over.

Early on, Aunt Colleen was a big part of our caregiving team. She was there two nights a week. She and Dad cooked dinner together, and then she would spend the night taking care of anything he needed during that time. A little over two years in, it just became too much for her. During one of our family check-ins, she said, "I think I'm at a point that if you find somebody you trust, I need to give up my nights." Of course, we found people who could cover her shift.

I knew that spending time with my dad was still very important to her (and to him), so we made sure that happened. On Saturdays, Dad and I would hit the gym and then pick up burgers and go spend a couple of hours with Aunt Colleen. We did that regularly to keep their relationship going and for she and I to have a chance to touch base, as well.

Be There for Each Other

The ability to listen to each other's needs was a really important key to keeping our family intact. Identifying your personality type, or who you are, and the personality types of the rest of your family members is helpful. Then being able to pull together as a joint effort, as with any team, is crucial. You must keep the goal in mind. The goal is to make caring for that person the priority, not getting our own way or having things done your way. This makes decision-making easier.

It also makes it easier to share the required grace. It makes it easier to put your faith and trust into the other people on the team. As I've talked about, this season will change the family dynamic. It's a whole different environment with different stressors. It's important to ensure that family relationships are nurtured through this process.

I talked about lunch with my sister and having that time to sit down and talk not just about Dad, but also about life. We started doing things for our own self-care together. Self-care wasn't a big thing for my sister. Being a life coach, I knew the importance of taking care of ourselves. We started doing things together to ensure that we were both getting the time for ourselves that we needed.

There was a salt room close to where Dad lived. Robin and I met there for an hour, simply to sit in a room that allows the salt to take the toxins out. We'd talk to each other about how we were doing. Being in town allowed me to engage in my sister's life during our caring season, which was important for our relationship.

Spending some weekend time there instead of at my farm, allowed me to go to her son's basketball games. Taking Dad to those ball games was great for him, but it was also great for my sister's and my relationship. Being able to spend time with his grandkids, building those relationships, was important for all of us. For my sister and me, we were actually more of a family in some ways than we had ever been as adults. I learned to understand Robin better as a person—what her needs were and how she thought, which always helps any relationship.

The more we think that everybody should be just like us, the less we get along.

I got to spend a lot of time with my aunt, hearing stories about what my dad's and her lives were like growing up. They had a lot of fun adventures. I learned things about Dad and her that I never knew. They were just two peas in a pod growing up. I had no idea that throughout their lives, they had been really close. Being able to honor that relationship and getting to know my aunt better was really a blessing in that season of time.

Since my dad's passing, I continue to make it a priority to go back to Kansas City and spend time with my sister, her family, and my aunt, to keep those relationships growing. I knew it would have to be something I was intentional about because relationships take time. When you take the opportunity that's given to you in these situations that aren't all that fun and make the best of them, one of the things that can happen is for those relationships to flourish.

When was the last time you intentionally invested in your relationships? There is a simple exercise that will be helpful for you to do to keep relationships a priority in this busy, stress-filled season.

- On a piece of paper, list those who are in this caregiving season with you.
- Rank how your caregiving season is impacting those relationships with numbers from one to ten—one being awful, I would rather not see them to ten, things have never been better.
- Record a "next step" to reconnect or communicate with each person on your list.

This seems like a really simple activity, but you will be surprised what taking the time to consider your relationships and write down a next step will do for you. While a notebook or any sheet of paper will do, I have also included a form in the back of this book for you to utilize.

Any time you can involve other people in the family, even if they would not be considered primary caregivers, it can help them to see the true dynamics of the situation. Robin's husband, John, was another person who was really supportive through the process. He would pick my dad up from the day-stay facility on Fridays. They would often hit the grocery store before John brought him home to me, where I would have dinner ready for him.

They had such adventures, not always fun ones, between the potty accidents and crazy behavior at times, but it brought John into what we were dealing with in a little way, bringing him into our daily world. He would tease and say he was Dad's chauffeur. I think that helped him to understand the stress of what was going on with Robin and me. It also helped me to appreciate how supportive he was of what we were doing for my dad.

Robin and John's children were always fun when around Grandpa. They were old enough to know there were things changing with him, but they were great with him during this season. Dad loved kids. It was fun to see him interact with them—especially my niece, Delaney. If Grandpa wouldn't come to the kitchen table, Delaney could always talk him into it. He had a soft spot for her. Even though the children were young, they were still a part of our team, and those relationships were so important.

Then, of course, my husband played a big role, too. With his farming, he wasn't able to spend the three days at my dad's with me very often, but the support he showed me was beyond measure. He was only a phone call away with his great advice and listening ear when I needed him. Any time he was with my dad, it was a joy to see them joke around and have a good time together. The whole team effort was all about everybody providing the support they could, in the role they were able to be in, and that was really important.

Caregiving can have a significant toll on romantic relationships. Sharing your struggles, joys, and concerns with your spouse will help them understand the juggle you are living out daily. But be aware of how your spouse is feeling and be sure to communicate your appreciation for his or her support. And, absolutely, prioritize time with your spouse.

You might find yourself in a position of caring for an aging parent while you still have children at home. There are lots of demands on your time, attention, and love. You will often feel torn and even think that no one is getting your best. The key is to help your children understand that elders have increased needs, and your family is going to be there to help. Ask your children what they would like to do to be a part of the team. It is just as important to get their buy-in as it is to get the buy-in from your parent.

As Robin's kids were during this time, your kids can be bright spots in the life of your loved one, offering smiles and the simple joys children bring. It is also important to remember you are setting the example for your kids of how to care for all family members and balance life's relationships, so be mindful of how well you are offering love and support to all members of your family.

We need to protect family relationships. It's important to know that those relationships can strengthen and grow into something even more special, if you give each other the grace and acceptance that are needed during this time. Caregiving doesn't always have to be a burden or a situation that tears the family apart. If we allow it, caregiving can be a vehicle for growth, for strength, and for building bigger and better relationships.

All challenges are opportunities for growth.

This was a big challenge in life—honoring Dad and making his last years as happy and healthy as possible. Through that challenge, I came out with improved relationships and opportunities to have memories and shared experiences that brought us all closer together.

Relating to the One Being Cared for

Let's come back to the parents for a moment as they are going through this season of change. Keeping this relationship intact is tough, but it has to be the priority. Dad and I were close. We had a really good relationship. Even through the years of caring for my mom, I was there to support my dad. I gave him breaks and spent time with my mom when he was playing softball a couple of times a week, trying to support him as much as I understood he needed in that season. My mom was nonverbal for about seven of the twelve years she had Alzheimer's. She didn't say anything that made sense and could only talk gibberish. I fed her, took her to the bathroom, bathed her; I took care of those physical needs for her.

My relationship with my dad was so different that I actually struggled with imagining what it would be like to do those things for my dad. I told my sister, "I don't think I can do that. I don't think I can see him in that way." When everything started, I wasn't sure at what point I would determine "I'm done. I can't do this anymore." Watching him change was difficult, and I thought the time would come when I would not feel comfortable taking care of him anymore.

The thing that was surprising to me was through his progression of the disease, I never felt uncomfortable with needing to take care of his physical needs. I just saw my dad as someone who couldn't do various things for himself, and because he couldn't do them for himself, I wasn't going to stand there and not help him. Just stepping in and taking care of what he couldn't do was a lot easier than I ever imagined.

I always saw my dad as someone who loved me more than anyone else, who had always been supportive, and had always been there for me, who was now in a place where he needed me. It was important to me to step in and meet those needs. Things were definitely difficult. He cussed. He hit. He was not kind, at times. But that wasn't really my dad. He was the epitome of a gentleman prior to the disease. I don't think I ever heard my dad cuss growing up. He played ball and served in the army, so I know he likely did, but he didn't use profanity in front of his girls until later in his disease. Hearing those things from his mouth was hard for my heart.

I knew somewhere inside, my daddy was there.

I still got those smiles, the pats on my arm or knee, and the hugs where he would hold on for a long while. He was the same person he had always been; he just was in a place where he was confused and things didn't make sense. It was hard on him. That helped me be able to step in and meet those needs.

I tried to remember how we had fun together before the disease. I tried to find things we could do together, things he would still enjoy. It helped that he was so competitive. I played volleyball in college so that was a love we shared. One of my favorite things was to go and play volleyball with him and the "senior" guys who played the pick up games he loved dearly. Dad had taken up volleyball after Mom passed away. It wasn't a sport he had played most of his life, but he sure enjoyed it later in life.

He also loved bowling. Oftentimes, I would schedule family time together, gathering the grandkids, my sister, her husband, and our aunt, and we'd all go bowling. When he would get a strike, he was so excited and had so much fun cheering everybody else on. I found those times that brought out my dad as much as possible; that was a big part of how I tried to keep that relationship alive. It's a process you'll discover as you go through it. In the thick of it, it's hard to remember the good times, but you have to in order to keep the relationship you have with your parent alive.

The process of going through an illness changes our parents enough. Creating pockets of comfort and normalcy, allowing them to be who they are and experience an enjoyable life even through the disease and corresponding changes, is so important. We kept him involved and active and having fun. As time progresses, it's going to get less and less fun, but finding those moments where you can still bring enjoyment and time everyone can share together, is important. It's not just for us but for our parent as well. It's about taking care of that relationship.

Dad was a thinker, and when he got to thinking and problem solving, you could see the anxiety in his face. When he was trying to figure out how to do something or what was wrong, keeping him in the moment of fun was helpful for his mental health, and it was amazing to experience that together. It's also okay to realize when something isn't fun.

The first year I was there, we planted bushes in the front of the house because it was time to refresh the yard. We worked together to do the planting and had a good afternoon dressing up the flowerbeds and making them look pretty. A year later, when it was time to refresh again, he wasn't near as helpful. He struggled with getting mud on his shoes and understanding how to dig the hole where it needed to be. He had not had a problem with the activity the year before. That was one of those moments when I realized that something we had done before might not happen again because it was causing Dad or me undue stress rather than bringing joy.

They are still the same people, but they likely need a little more help now than ever before.

The lesson is to do what you can, while you can! Make the best of it when times are good and when they're not, understand that it's part of the process. My dad was still my dad; he was just in a place where he needed more help than he ever had during my life. Understanding this perspective will help you keep the relationship with your loved one intact for as long as possible.

When Your Relationship is Strained

I understand that not everyone has a good relationship with their parents or their siblings. That is not my experience. My childhood was full of consistency, love, and support. Of course, no one's life is perfect, but I am blessed to have many more good memories than bad. But that might not be your story. It might be incredibly hard for you to imagine partnering with your sibling or even caring for your aging parents. That is okay. Your story does not have to look like mine.

I do want you to consider what you want your story to look like, though. Years from now, what will you regret? Don't allow past hurts to dictate what the future looks like. Finding healing and forgiveness for your parents will make you a better parent and person.

> *There is no simple fix to those difficult relationships*
> *with even more difficult people.*
> —Michele Howe, *Caring for Our Aging Parents*

Caring for someone who did not do a good job of caring for you when you were growing up has to be one of the most challenging things you will do. Relationships are complicated, and they require a large dose of forgiveness, grace, and patience. It might take some outside support for you to explore how to find what will be required of you to care for them as they age. But do it; I know you won't regret it.

Your relationship might be broken to the point that you aren't the only one who needs to forgive. You can't control someone else's feelings; all you can do is the best you can to repair the relationship. If you and your parent trigger each other, then being a part of the hands-on caring team won't be the best idea, but that doesn't mean you do nothing to support them. You can still be a part of the team.

Maybe you find yourself at odds with your siblings and that makes caring for your parent challenging. Having difficult conversations can help. Be willing to talk about your differences; find forgiveness, and gather around your parents to support them.

The source of many sibling conflicts comes from a few places according to Carolyn Rosenblatt in *The Family Guide to Aging Parents*. She states that lifelong behavioral patterns will still exist and are frequently the root cause of conflicts. Just because your parent needs you in a way they haven't before doesn't mean a happy family will magically come together to support them.

Rosenblatt goes on to recommend communicating in advance of the parent's need to help control the conflict. Identify one sibling to take the leadership role, whether it's for a specific period of time or over a specific project, can take the headache out of this season. She also recommends bringing in professional help. If your family is one in frequent conflict, you don't have to go it alone. Outside, objective professionals can help everyone realistically plan for the current and future needs of your parent.

Notes

_____

_____

_____

_____

_____

_____

_____

_____

_____

_____

_____

_____

_____

_____

_____

_____

_____

_____

Dear Confused Daughter/Son,

It is okay to not have all the answers; no one knows everything about everything.

There are many resources at your disposal, and you can support your parent in just the way he/she needs. Rely on others' perspectives and insights to learn what you need to know.

You have what it takes to search for answers to the challenges you and your family are facing in this caring season.

Rayna

CHAPTER 4

Know What You Don't Know

W hen walking into any new season of life, you typically don't know what to expect. Let's say you're a newlywed. Many questions may rise to the surface of your thoughts. What is it going to be like to live with someone in your space all the time and have to make joint decisions you've never had to make before? Moving into this season of caring for an aging parent is full of many unknowns. It's a season where you will often find yourself saying, "I didn't even know I needed to know that."

All of this information quickly becomes overwhelming. One of the things that comes to mind, as I think about it all, is the medical terminology you are about to be inundated with. Watching a parent try to negotiate Medicare, other insurances, doctors' appointments, and medications comes with this job. There are so many things you and your parents need to understand as you start this journey, which is why I am sharing my journey with you.

As my dad was progressing through his disease, one of the struggles we faced was with doctors. We needed them to be a part of our team. Usually my sister and I attended doctors' appointments with Dad. We reached a time when we had a doctor that was supposed to be in charge of his medication for the Alzheimer's specifically. Those prescriptions included anti-depressants for the behavioral consequences or by-products of being overwhelmed with a lack of understanding about what's going on in his environment.

The Doctor Isn't Always Right

Dad was frustrated, and he wasn't behaving like himself. We called the doctor's office and had left messages, but we weren't getting return calls. Finally, they called in a prescription, and we picked it up. Lo and behold, one of the warnings on the medication was to avoid using with people with dementia. It literally said, *can cause sudden death.* That's a pretty scary thing to read as you are dispensing that pill to your father who is experiencing dementia. Thankfully, we saw it in time and unfortunately, we received no explanation from the doctor.

We held off on giving Dad that medication until we scheduled an appointment and went in and spoke with her. I walked out of that appointment still feeling like she had not fully answered my questions about why she had chosen to use that drug, especially when there was the possibility of a major side effect. She never explained why we couldn't try something else. I just didn't feel satisfied with the answers.

As my sister and I were talking about it, we decided to look around and see what else was available. We contacted a couple of neurologists closer to home to ask about making a transfer of his care to someone else. My sister attended a couple of meetings with the new neurologist group and had some conversations with them.

One of the things that really bothered us was that Dad was still on three different Alzheimer's medications. At that time, in the research on Alzheimer's, the only available medications were targeted for the early stages of the disease. But we were nine years into my dad's diagnosis, well beyond the early stages. We looked at these prescription medications, thinking, "Why is he still taking these?"

We asked the neurologist this question and were told, "Oh, you don't want to take him off of those. I had one patient whom I took off of the medication, and her behavior just went haywire. It was a really bad situation." But when we pushed for more info, when we asked what it was doing for our dad, we couldn't get answers. We needed to know what the benefit of him taking these drugs was, and yet, we couldn't get a straight answer. Once again, we made the decision that this wasn't the right doctor for us and went looking for a different physician. Thankfully, we did find somebody who could have conversations with us, who helped us understand what he was taking and why. It is very important to follow your gut. You have to take the time to do the research and understand. And if you can't get your questions answered, you probably don't have the right people on your team.

If you don't feel that your loved one's doctor is on your team, it's time to find a new team member.

I think sometimes we get so used to just doing what doctors tell us. I'm not sure why we think they're always right. All of us are human. We make mistakes, no matter what our job is. There are no perfect people—even doctors. Doctoring is a process of understanding symptoms and following protocols. There is a very distinct methodology they follow when prescribing medication.

The key is, there are no two people exactly alike who process medications exactly the same, just like there are no two children who learn to read exactly the same way. We're different, distinct individuals, and each patient handles medications differently. Doctors are doing the best they can, but they're not necessarily the only people with the solutions. It's important to understand this as we step in to advocate for our parents. You are your parent's voice.

If the current doctor is not the right one, then it's okay to go look for someone else. Sometimes, we feel a loyalty to a specific doctor. *Oh, Dad's been with him for twenty-five years.* Well, that doesn't mean he's ready to deal with my dad at this stage of his life. Geriatrics is a specialized area of practice, and there aren't a lot of doctors in this specialization. Finding doctors who are willing to research new things and listen can be quite impactful to the overall health of your mom or dad. Our medical care today is compartmentalized. My dad had a cardiologist; he had a neurologist; he had a urologist; he had an oncologist; and he had a primary care physician. He had all of these different specialists, but they never talked to each other. They didn't sit around a table and have a conversation about my dad.

One thing that we found helpful was a primary care physician who was willing to sit down and talk with us and really look at all of his medical reports in an effort to understand everything that was happening with all the specialists. She was willing to have conversations with us, helping us reach an understanding about what they were telling us and how his overall health was impacting each of those areas.

There was a point in time when Dad's doctor took him off of one of the early stage Alzheimer's medications, and my dad's blood pressure dropped dramatically. He started passing out. It was very scary. We had no idea what was happening, but being able to talk to his primary care physician and telling her what was happening gave us relief. She talked us through the different symptoms that could happen from certain medications and helped us get to a quick discovery of what was happening. Come to find out, my dad was on three high blood pressure medications because the Alzheimer's medications caused his blood pressure to be so elevated. Three weeks after removing one Alzheimer's medication, my dad was off of two of the three high blood pressure medications. High blood pressure was not something he struggled with during the last two years of his life because we were able to remove those medications.

*There are many intricate pieces involved
in the care of someone who is aging.*

As a layperson, you can't know everything, but you do need to have someone who can help explain everything at the right times and who will take the time to work within your team. In fact, Dad's primary care physician did make a phone call to the cardiologist explaining what we were seeing. They put their heads together and came up with some strategies to try. Getting those team members on the same page and having someone who could explain it to us in layman's terms while using medical jargon with a peer was beneficial to us. The last two years of my dad's life was considerably better because we had a primary care physician (PCP) that listened to us and communicated with the other doctors.

Advocating for Our Loved Ones

Being your loved one's advocate is one of the most important roles you will play as a family caregiver. When someone is in the middle of a medical crisis, the brain is overwhelmed with all of the things happening to them, whether it is pain, fear, or any other emotions that creep up. All of those feelings and thoughts are paralyzing to the brain. The logical side of the brain can't engage as easily when it's under that kind of strain. When we're watching our parents struggle and having concerns, we will have emotional reactions, but we are still one step removed, allowing us to be an advocate in a clear, calm fashion when our parents can't be.

While stepping into that advocacy role, you have to be gracious with your parents. You can't step over them; you can't talk over them. You can't be the only voice, unless you have a situation like mine, where my dad eventually lost his voice because he wasn't able to communicate his needs any longer. This comes back to relationship. It's important to walk alongside and advocate in a way that is respectful to your parent. And you'll want to make sure your parent still has a voice as long as they're able to have that voice. I think we all need advocates at different seasons of our lives and aging is definitely a season where we need that advocate to step forward and be there for us.

Non-Traditional Treatments

There may be reasons and times you want to step out of the traditional way of handling challenges. You'll need doctors who are willing to let you try some of those out-of-the-box ideas. Dad's PCP suggested some alternatives to regular medications, so we did try non-traditional treatments.

One of the most amazing ideas was called an ionic footbath detox. There is a lot of research that supports both sides as far as whether it works or not. After his doctor mentioned this idea of taking my dad to have footbaths, I investigated the process. Robin and I decided it was worth a try. An iconic foot detox pulls the toxins out of your body through your feet. This practice required us to take Dad to soak his feet in a special bath for a short period of time. After six treatments, it was amazing to witness the clarity my dad seemed to gain.

He was able to create some new memories, and he seemed to have more lucidity in conversations. It didn't necessarily make him more able to handle the everyday frustrations, but with that clarity came more calmness. It was amazing to see the difference that something as simple as a foot detox could make for him. We also used a lot of vitamins and mineral supplements. B12 can help feed the brain things that it might be missing, so we tried some B12 shots. We found some improvement for my dad as far as his overall ability to think a bit more clearly in situations.

There are a lot of non-traditional things out there. Just like with medication, they don't all work for everyone, but if you can help alleviate some of the pain or give your parent a few moments of clarity, it is well worth your time to do the research. In taking that time, we found natural options to prescription medications. Two of the benefits of those natural options are fewer side effects and interactions with other medications.

With any new medication or treatment introduced into the system, you have to be able to stop and question: *What is the benefit and what could the side effects be?* Oftentimes, we find older people are on the same prescriptions for years. Most doctors are not comfortable taking someone off of a medication that another doctor prescribed. So even if the patient isn't still experiencing the struggle or symptom they had when the medication was prescribed, they continue to take it. It can be a challenge to understand the reasons and side effects of medications, not to mention making sure everybody on the medical team is on the same page.

Active Advocacy

Doctor Jennifer Ashton stated on "Good Morning America" that we all need to be active patients, and I think that's true. In this role, you may not be the patient, but you need to be an active advocate. She recommended asking these basic questions:

- What are the risks of doing this?
- What are the risks of not doing this?
- What are the benefits of doing this?
- What are the benefits of not doing this?

So, even with the natural or alternative options, you still have to ask what risks exist. What are the benefits? Does one outweigh the other? We found multiple natural treatments with my dad—from CBD oil for anxiety to magnesium to keep his bowel movements regular, and from ionic foot detoxes to regular massages. There were a lot of things we felt helped keep his quality of life at the highest level possible.

The goal is happy and healthy as long as possible.

Doctors can be more focused on the cure than the care. This is one of the most challenging obstacles. There is an underlying difference in our thought processes—as a daughter and a doctor. Doctors have been trained, and they've invested their lives in learning their practice. Their ultimate goal is to cure. For example, they want blood pressure under control. Or with heart surgery, they've been able to do the bypasses and move the heart to a healthier state than it was before. The "cure only" perspective is to push, push, push, and do what needs to be done to reach the cure or save a life, but sometimes, the cure is worse than the disease.

Finding common ground on the same page with the physician and reaching the understanding that yes, we wanted him cured as much as possible, but we also wanted him to have the best quality of life that was available to him right then was invaluable.

As an example, Dad developed a quarter-sized spot of melanoma on his collarbone. Melanoma is a cancer that can be nasty, even deadly if left untreated. In fact, if not caught early, most forms of it are not curable. They can do surgery and remove it, but as far as using che-motherapy and radiation to cure the actual melanoma cancer cells, it's not something the medical community has been very successful with.

We were about nine years into Dad's Alzheimer's diagnosis when the melanoma diagnosis surfaced. At this point, Dad was not able to live alone or drive any longer, but Aunt Colleen was there with him. We knew we weren't curing the Alzheimer's, and we had to decide exactly what were we going to put him through in treating this cancer. We opted for the surgery to remove it, and thankfully, it had not spread. Our doctor was very surprised.

One of the things I loved about the oncologist we worked with is that he understood my dad's Alzheimer's diagnosis. Over the five years that he monitored my dad's cancer (or lack of), one of the things that he talked to us about frequently was that melanoma often goes to the lungs or to the brain.

While we did the testing to see if it was in the lungs, the doctor gave us the choice and recommended that it was not smart to put our dad through an MRI every six months or every year to see if the melanoma had gone to his brain. There was nothing we could do about it if it had moved to that location. He knew that my sister and I didn't want to treat it through any aggressive measures if it was found in the brain. I appreciated him sharing other options, even though most were not going to work for us in our situation, which included my dad's age and other diagnoses.

Find doctors, like this one, that really hone in on what you want as a family.

I have enjoyed reading the book, *Being Mortal: Medicine and What Matters in the End.* The author is Atul Gawandea, a practicing surgeon who reveals the struggles that doctors have with death. He mentions that the patient's anxiety about his own struggle with death affects how the doctor talks with the patient about the possibility of death. He recommends a new approach in talking with patients, making sure that doctors are listening and asking questions, such as, "What are their goals? What are their priorities? What do they need to understand?"

He states that because doctors are uncomfortable discussing patients' anxieties about death, they fall back on false hopes and treatments, which are actually shortening lives instead of improving them. It was an interesting read, seeing these circumstances from the perspective of a doctor who ultimately realized that his goal is always to cure, but that goal might not always be in the best interest of the patient. Again, having these difficult conversations, in an effort to make sure that everyone is on the same page, is very important.

> *The ultimate goal is not a good death but a good life*
> *—all the way to the very end.*
> —Atul Gawandea

The Alzheimer's Association research has found that less than fifty percent of the people diagnosed with Alzheimer's had been told they have the disease. That's mind boggling to me! So fifty percent of the people that have it don't even know their diagnosis. After hearing this, I took a moment to step back and remember how my mom was diagnosed in 1986. Mom and Dad decided to have specific testing done to check her memory, as it had become obvious that she was having problems with it.

When the doctor, who was a general practitioner, talked to my parents about the results, he let them know there were some concerns, but they just needed to see how things progressed. After that conversation, he sent them home with a folder that included the paperwork from the test results. When my dad looked through it, the diagnosis of Alzheimer's was there. My mom was fifty-three years old. That doctor's discomfort with giving my mom a terminal diagnosis interfered with the way he spoke to my parents, excluding critical information about where Mom was and what was happening with her.

We had a similar experience when my dad was diagnosed. His first diagnosis, in 2003, was "mild cognitive impairment." What that means is there are some memory issues, but they are not significant enough to interfere with daily living tasks. Through monitoring with a neurologist and repeated visits, they continued to watch (and assess) him vigilantly.

In 2006, an assistant pulled my dad in to do some neurological testing while the doctor took my sister, aunt, and me to a different room to ask us the routine questions. This was a different doctor then the one we had been seeing. She started the conversation with, "Well, we know with Alzheimer's, this is expected . . ." And she just kept on talking. That's how we found out my dad had crossed from mild cognitive impairment to Alzheimer's. It was devastating to our family to hear that diagnosis, much less have it dropped into a conversation as if we already knew. It was horrible.

Doctors Are Human Too

Sometimes, we lose the perspective that doctors are human too, and not all of them are comfortable talking about these diagnoses with their patients. It's important to be proactive in how you approach the doctor to say what you need from them, whether it's to give it to you straight, to be sure they are clear so that you understand what is going on, or to approach the communication of hard truths softly. You need to give the medical team the freedom to be open with you, possibly designating someone as the medical advocate so the doctors know which one they can disclose the full details to.

There are many reasons to keep the lines of communication fully open with the doctors. This is also true when it comes to medication. When we found the general practitioner that really spent the time with us and invested in us as a family, Dad was on fourteen different prescription medications. When she saw his prescription list, she was concerned. She explained that once people move beyond four prescriptions, there are various interactions and side effects and oftentimes, the patient is not getting the full impact of the medication.

Consider our example of how taking away the one early-stage Alzheimer's medication impacted Dad's blood pressure. One of the side effects of that drug is increased blood pressure. Dad was on three different medications to counteract the side effect of that one medication. This is why it's so important to understand what the benefits and risks of the prescriptions are and also to know how they will affect the overall life of the person who is taking them.

When we get any prescription package, it usually comes with what seems like pages of adverse effects or reactions that can happen from taking that particular medication. It's overwhelming. There's so much to decipher on there.

Your pharmacist can be a huge advocate, looking for interactions that are negative but not necessarily easy to see.

Each body metabolizes medications differently. Both my mom and dad were very sensitive to prescription medication, so we knew to keep an eye out for the side effects that could be a problem. We always asked that they take a lower dose initially to see if they would get the benefit the doctors were looking for with less chance of problems.

We also navigated the lowering of doses to see if we were ready to take Dad off some medications. We worked with the doctors as we tried the natural options I talked about earlier because we felt they were more beneficial to him and his quality of life, reducing the negative side effects that all of those different prescription medications caused.

There is a reason that medication is prescribed the way it is, and it's important to pay attention and follow the directions.

I know medication management can be very overwhelming and frightening for someone who's not experienced this before. As you work to help someone manage their medicine, you might find that medications are being taken at the wrong time. For example, they should be taking a pill twice a day, and instead, they're taking two pills at one time.

So Many Meds

In an earlier chapter, I talked about knowing the different strengths and weaknesses of the people on your team. My sister is an accountant—into the details and able to put together the best medication list I've ever seen. It included the name of the prescription, whether it was the generic or the name brand, when it should have been taken, what the dosage was, how many pills there were (i.e.: one pill, half a pill, two pills). This list also included a description of the pill.

This detailed summary is important because if you've ever managed someone's prescriptions, putting them into a.m. and p.m. pillboxes and that pillbox falls, it creates a giant mess. Sometimes, you might have your prescriptions in the pillbox, and you run into an issue and the doctor says, let's take them off "this" and put them on "that" instead. Having that physical description is very helpful in making it easy to identify which pill is which.

With a simple glance at that medication list, where my sister had written *tiny yellow tablet with 81 on it* made it much simpler to find. We also listed where it was purchased from, what it was prescribed for, and the name of the prescribing doctor. And then we had details in another column, such as when he started taking it, if he had any side effects, or if there had been any changes. For instance, if we reduced a dose from 500 milligrams to 250 milligrams, the date and the reason for the change was documented right there. We had meds listed as a.m. or p.m. This was so useful, not only for our caregiving team but also for our doctors. We had all the doctor's names, phone numbers, and contact information so we could pick up the phone at any time and discuss any concerns.

I have a list that looks like this for myself. I'm not on a lot of prescription medications, but I take vitamins and other supplements. When I walk into the doctor's office, I can hand them my list of medications and say, "This is what I take, why I take it, when I take it, and how long I've been taking it." This is something I recommend not only for caregiving but also for you.

A complete and accurate medication list is the foundation for addressing medication management issues.

Being able to manage medication is an important piece of caregiving. Medicine names are long and complicated. Being able to keep track of them and knowing what kind of side effects you might be looking for if they're starting something new is important. It is also helpful to have them all listed in one place when you want to talk to the doctor about how any new medication they put them on might impact another prescription they are on. Whether it is an antibiotic for an infection or something new that needs to be introduced, being able to have prescription information at your fingertips and have conversations with the doctors can make a big difference. Be sure to share this information with any caregiver who is administering medications, as well.

MEDICATIONS TAKEN DAILY

Date Of Birth: ___ As Of: 1/27/17 Printed: 10/19/20

Medication	Time	Dosage	Pill	Description Of Pill	Purchased From / Prescription #	Condition	Doctor	Started Taking	Status
Aspirin	AM	81 MG	1	tiny yellow tablet w/ 81	Hy-Vee	Heart		2000; Stopped 5 Days Prior To Surgery on 8/13/13; Resumed 9/2013; 10/23/16 - Reduced to 2x's/Week (M & Th); 10/25/16 - **Increased back to daily**	
Finasteride (Generic for Proscar)	AM	2.5 mg (1/2 tablet)	0.5	small round blue tablet w/F5	Hy-Vee	Prostate		3/19/2007; 10/31/16 - Dr. Wilson advised not to reduce due to extremely enlarged prostate; 11/08/16 - **Reduce to 1/2**	
Divalproex Sodium (Generic for Depakote)	AM	250 mg	1	medium oblong light pink tablet	Hy-Vee	Anti-Depression / Anti-Anxiety		3/22/16 w/250mg (Replaced Celexa); 6/15/16 - Increased to 1 1/2 Tablets (375mg); 7/26/16 - Increased to 500mg; 11/8/16 - **Reduced to 250mg**	
Rivastigmine (Generic For Exelon) – Patch	AM	9.5 mg–24 hr patch	-	skin colored patch	Hy-Vee	Memory		9/15/2008 (rotate back and front placement); 3/24/16 - Increased from 9.5 to 13.3 and switched to generic; 10/25/16 - Reduced from 13.3 back to 9.5; **Stopped 2/20/17**	Stopped
Quetiapine Fumarate (Generic for Seroquel)	AM	12.5mg (1/2 tablet)	0.5	tiny round coral tablet	Hy-Vee	Anxiety		3/3/14 - Added AM dose; 8/22/14 - Stopped AM Dose; 8/29/14 - Added back AM Dose; 3/14/16 - Increased to 1 full pill; 6/8/16 - Cut Back To 1/2; **01/27/17 - Stop**	
Chlorthalidone	AM	12.5mg (1/2 tablet)	0.5	small oblong white tablet	Hy-Vee	Water Pill / Blood Pressure		9/12/15 (Replaced HCTZ); 10/31/16 - **Reduced to 1/2 dose; Hold when BP <120; 11/8/16 - HOLD**	
Valsartan	AM	160 MG (1/2 tablet)	0.5	large irregular shaped mauve tablet	Hy-Vee	Blood Pressure		9/12/15 (Replaced Losartan); 11/03/16 - **Reduced to 1/2 dose (320 to 160); Hold when BP < 110; 11/8/16 - HOLD**	
Saffron	AM		1	medium light coral capsule	Hy-Vee	Agitation		Started 10/13/16; Stop 1/2/17	
K-PAX Energy	AM		1	large brown speckled tablet	O'Brien Pharmacy	Multi-Vitamin + Digestion		Started 10/23/16; Hold 11/06/16; Restarted 11/15/16; Hold 11/22/16 - Trouble taking pills	
CF Joint Care	AM		1	large peach capsule	O'Brien Pharmacy	Arthritis		Started 10/23/16 (Replaced ibuprofen); Must be opened and taken in applesauce	
Metanx	AM		1	medium circle purple tablet		Brain Health		11/03/16 - AM Dose - Replaced Bioavailable Folate	
MitoQ	AM	5mg	1	medium tan & white capsule		Energy/Brain Health		Started 11/15/16	
Relax Day	AM		1	large white capsule		Agitation		Started 1/1/17	
MCT Oil	AM	1 tsp	-	clear liquid	Vitacost.com	Brain Health		Started 1/16/17	
Clindamycin	AM		1	medium blue capsule	Hy-Vee	Infection		Started AM Dose 10/25/16; Hold 11/06/16; Restarted 11/15/16; Hold 12/17/16; Restarted 12/26/16; 1/1/17 - HOLD	Stop
B-12	AM	100	1x / week	injection - red liquid	Stark Pharmacy	Memory		Started 10/22/16	

9 Medicines

7 + 1/2 + Oil + Shot

Medication	Time	Dosage	Pill	Description Of Pill	Purchased From / Prescription #	Condition	Doctor	Started Taking	Status
Quetiapine Fumarate (Generic for Seroquel)	3:00 PM	12.5mg (1/2 tablet)	0.5	tiny round coral tablet	Hy-Vee	Anxiety		12/10/2013; Switched from 4:00 to 3:00 2/27/14; 3/14/16 Increased to 1 full pill; 6/25/16 - Decreased to 1/2	Stop

Medicine	Time	Dose	Qty	Description	Purpose	Source	Notes	Stop
Fluconazole	PM		1	medium oblong tan tablet	Yeast	Hy-Vee	Started 10/22/16, Hold 11/05/16; Restarted 12/31/16 (AM and PM for 5 Days)	
Iodoral	Monday 3:00 PM	12.5	1	medium oblong tan tablet	Iodine	Hy-Vee	Started /2/17	
3 Medicines			2 + 1/2					
Vitamin D3	PM	1000 IU	1	medium round white tablet	General Health / Memory	Vitacost.com	1/13/' 1	
Alaskol	PM	25 MG (1/2 tablet)	0.5	small round white tablet wnGc 293	Heart	916442	Since Before 10/25/00 - Moved Back To Evening 1/25/06; 5/11/14 - Reduced dosage to 1/2 pill. 11/07/16 - HOLD	
Amlodipine	PM	2.5 MG (1/2 tablet)	0.5	medium round white tablet ~54.771	Blood Pressure	a42305	9/2/2009 10/31/16 - Moved to PM: 1 /02/16 - Reduced from 5 MG to 2.5 MG (1/2 Tablet); 11/03/16 - Stopped due to low nighttime BP	
Flora 20-14 Ultra Strength	PM	1 Capsule	1	small oblong white capsule	Probiotic / Digestion	Vitacost.com	3/7/16 - Replaced Pro-X10	
Claritin	PM	10mg	1	small white oblong tablet	Allergies / Congestion	Hy-Vee	Switched from Zyrtec; 4/13/15, 11/7/16 - Hold	
Senna-S	PM	50mg + 8.6mg	1	medium orange tablet	Constipation (Laxative + Stool Softner)	Amazon	Started 3/10/2016 (Replaced Miralax)	
Tolterodine Tartrate (Generic for Detrol LA)	PM	4 mg	1	medium oblong light green capsule w/2	Bladder	Hy-Vee	2/29/2008 - 4mg, 1/14/16 - Decreased To 2mg Capsule; 2/25/17- Increase back to 4mg and move to PM	
Divalproex Sodium (Generic for Depakote)	PM	250 mg	4	medium oblong light pink tablet	Anti-Depression / Anti-Anxiety	992677	Started 3/22/16 w/250mg (Replaced Zelexa); 6/25/16 - Increased to 375mg; 7/26/16 - Increased to 500mg; 9/27/16 - Increased to 750; 10/13/16 - Decreased to 500; 11/7/16 HOLD; 11/8/16 - Decrease to 250mg; 12/30/1 - HOLD	
Quetiapine Fumarate (Generic for Seroquel)	PM	12.5mg (1/2 tablet)	0.5	tiny round-spiral tablet	Anxiety	Hy-Vee	10/13/16 - Added 1/2 pill. ~1/06/16 - Stopped	
Clindamycin	PM		1	medium blue/green capsule	Infection	Hy-Vee	Started PM Dose 10/22/16; Hold 11/05/16	Stop
K-PAX Energy	PM		1	large brown speckled tablet	Multi-Vitamin - Digestion	O'Brien Pharmacy	Started 10/22/16; Hold 11/05/16	Stop
CF Joint Care	PM		1	large peach capsule	Arthritis	O'Brien Pharmacy	Started 10/22/16 (Replaced Ibuprofen); Must be opened and taken in applesauce	
Metanx	PM		1	medium circle purple tablet	Sleep / Digestion	Amazon	Started PM Dose 11/2/16 (Repla-ed Bioavailable Folate)	
Magnesium & Potassium Aspartate	PM	300mg & 99mg	1	large white oblong capsule	Sleep / Digestion	Amazon	Started 12/30/16; Must be opened and taken in applesauce	
CBD Oil	PM	1 drop with medicated cream		oil	Agitation	bluebird botanicals	Include several drops in with the cream for his back	
Pain Cream	PM				Pain	Stark Pharmacy	Rub on lower back	
Levofloxacin	PM		1	large oblong tan tablet	Infection	Hy-Vee	Started 11/5/16 - 10 Days (Last dose 1/14/16 PM); Started 12/16/16 - 10 Days (Last dose 12/25/16 PM)	
9 Medicines				7 + Cream + Oil				

When it comes to doing research on medications, it can get very complicated. You need to understand as much as you can by asking questions as you go. Here are some starters:

- Why is this the best option?
- What benefits will this medication bring to quality of life?
- What are typical issues with this medication?
- How might a reaction look?
- What kind of things do we need to be aware of?
- What happens if this doesn't go well?

Learn, in layman terms, the best you can about each drug. Neither my sister nor I had any medical background. If you have a nurse in the family, that's a great thing. Have them take a look at it as well; they're going to be able to decipher a lot of the stuff that might be over your head. But if you are like us and don't have that option, ask every question you can think of so you understand the best you can.

And let's not forget that pills are not the only form that medications can come in. It's more than just handing patients a few pills and something to wash them down with. Be aware and if you find that there is difficulty in administering or taking the medication as prescribed, ask the pharmacist, "Is there another option available?"

With Alzheimer's, swallowing pills can be difficult, especially when you have a lot and have to do it frequently; getting liquid forms of medications became helpful. Knowing what pill is okay to crush and what pill is not okay to crush is crucial. Can you mix the medications in applesauce or in yogurt or in a small quantity of peanut butter to eat with a meal? There were lots of different tricks we found, which made giving medications to my dad much easier.

There's an Alzheimer's medication that is administered through the skin on a patch that you change daily. It is imperative that you take the old patch off when you put the new one on. There have been incidences of sudden death due to overdose by having too many patches on at the same time. All medications have specific instructions on how they should be administered and sometimes when they should be administered.

Ensure you're tracking and administering them appropriately and ask the questions when you run into a challenge. Ask the questions because there are definitely lots of options. You will be able to help your parent much more as you ask questions and become more aware.

Dear Grieving Daughter/Son,

Watching a parent near the end of his or her life is one of the most difficult things you will ever do. There is no getting ready for the goodbye. No matter how much you feel prepared for them to go, it will still surprise you.

You will not regret being intentional with the time you have with your parent. It will be heartbreaking to watch, and grief is to be expected along to way. There is hope you will find peace again.

Rayna

CHAPTER 5

Walking Them Home

I've talked about treatments and about doctor care and about medications and their management. But what about the tough topic of *end of life*? The discomfort cannot stop us from learning what we need to know to be able to walk our parent home well.

Death planning is an uncomfortable topic because number one, we don't want to lose our loved ones. Number two, we don't want to think about our own mortality, but the truth is none of us are getting out of here alive. We have to be willing to understand that death is part of the journey that we're all on.

There are many pieces to be aware of. One of the hardest pieces to deal with is the legality of it all. You need to ensure that you have your legal ducks in a row. Most people have heard of a durable power of attorney, and I believe that no matter your age, you need to have a durable power of attorney. This is a document that gives someone you can trust the right to be able to speak on your behalf if you can't do it for yourself. With a durable power of attorney, the document's language states an agent's authority applies if you become incapacitated.

It is important to realize there are two types of powers of attorney. You don't have to designate the same person to handle your money and take care of your physical needs. You can have two different people step into those roles. A medical power of attorney is a legal document that names one person the health care agent of another person. Your agent has the ability to make health care decisions on your behalf. This document can be used if it is determined by a doctor that you are incapable of making such decisions or you are unable to communicate your wishes.

You cannot assume that just because you're married, your spouse will be automatically designated as the person who can speak for you if you were unable to speak for yourself during any kind of medical situation.

All states are different. If you find yourself in a situation where your loved one is incapacitated, and you step in and say, "I'm the spouse. I'm the one who will make the decisions concerning his care," all should be fine unless someone protests. It could be a child or another relative who steps in to protest your decisions. I'm in the state of Kansas, and if there is a situation where the power of attorney is challenged, the hospital will convene a panel that will make the final decision. By getting that durable power of attorney for your financials and the medical durable power of attorney for the medical decisions made on your behalf, you will save a lot of pain if a situation arises where they need to be enforced.

One of the challenges we ran into was with understanding what constitutes a life-saving measure. We have all watched television shows that incorporated ventilators and CPR, and they are obviously used as life-saving measures. But in reality, it's a really broad term. These measures could be applied in different ways and in different situations. If I'm in a car accident tomorrow, I might want you to go ahead and maintain my life for a little bit longer to see if I'm going to recover or just see what other options are available. If I'm eighty-five years old, and I have Alzheimer's disease and am involved in a car accident, that's not the same situation because the chance of recovery or getting even close to the same quality of life before the accident is not the same.

It's important to know what end of life means and what the actual lifesaving measures mean. I was surprised when my mom had a psychotic break that caused her to not be able to leave this cycle of talking and screaming. The end of her life was very difficult. We took her to the hospital, and they did numerous tests but couldn't find what was causing this cycle. As time went on, she was less and less able to perform daily tasks due to the cycle. The doctors eliminated all the things they could think of that might have caused this behavior. They tried different medications, but they just couldn't stop this cycle for my mom. She could no longer eat or walk.

We reached a point where we had to accept there was nothing that could be done for her and we had to let her go. We needed to know what that looked like. I was shocked to find out that IV fluids are considered life-saving measures. Oxygen can be considered a life-saving measure. Blood pressure medication can be a life-saving measure. It's a lot more complicated than I, as a layperson, realized. Taking IV fluids from my mom meant stopping the medications they were giving her that were being administered through the IV because those medications weren't available in a format for someone who was not able to swallow.

This choice limited the things we were able to do for her at the end of her life. So it's important to have these conversations with your loved ones and understand where their heart is on this situation. End of life care is not really interchangeable with life-saving measures. You need to know what they really want you to do (and not do) for them. It does make for a tough conversation, but it's a lot easier to make those decisions at the end of life when you're confident that you understand what the person really wants, even when they can't tell you.

At this point, hospice was not an option for our family. With the information and council of the experts at hospice, I think our family's experience of losing my mom would have been different. A good hospice team will help facilitate the conversations for your family. I want to challenge you to not wait until hospice comes in to have the conversations, though. Start learning what you need to know now to support your parents at the end of their lives.

From state to state, rules and regulations for end of life are different. Even in doctors' minds, what a lifesaving measure is can be different from one medical professional to another. There is a lot of gray area, so you want to be confident in the decisions you will have to make. I'm a fighter; if you tell me it can't be done, I'm going to prove you wrong. One of the things I prayerfully considered while caring for my dad was, *when do I stop fighting?* That was a hard, hard question for me. It was something I knew would go against the grain of who I am. So I prayed, "Lord, help me know when it's time to stop fighting for my dad."

Prayer is a great way to find peace.

Dad was doing well and there wasn't anything that would make us think he was going to be gone within a month. The beginning of the end came when he had a blood clot that developed in his leg, and he had surgery to have that clot removed because it was causing extreme pain for him. The only thing that would ease that pain was to get the blood circulation back to his leg.

He did really well with the surgery. We were not sure what to expect after surgery with his advanced Alzheimer's. It was difficult in the hospital. He experienced a lot of confusion, but we kept all of our caregivers in place, and my sister and I were there. He continued to see the faces he recognized; we knew the tricks of how to help him best after surgery.

After his stay in the hospital, he was discharged to a rehab facility where they were able to work with him on being able to walk again. During the surgery to remove the blood clot, they also opened up a couple inches on both sides of the calf to allow for the swelling that naturally happens when blood flows again. Those large incisions were open wounds that went all the way to the muscle, and that's where the problem started.

We saw some unusual things with one of the wounds; it wasn't healing well. Despite that, we were able to get him to his house. Dad was even able to walk a hundred feet at the rehab facility the day they released him.

We had set up a nice, little space downstairs for us as caregivers to be right there with him. He had access to a bathroom and having him set up there would make it easy for him to continue his in-home physical therapy. He was in good spirits. You could tell he knew he was home once we got him settled in there.

On the sixth morning of him being home, I prayed my normal prayer, "Lord, help me to let go when it's time to let go."

God said, "It's time."

I was shocked. I thought, "Well, Lord, you didn't understand my prayer. You must have that wrong."

And He said, "No, Rayna, it's time to stop fighting." I struggled with that, but as I looked at my dad while sitting with him by his bedside, I saw that he was done fighting. There was just a change that morning from the day before.

There was a peace that came over him.

That afternoon, the daily visiting in home care nurse arrived to look at the wounds, and she pulled my sister aside because I happened to be out for a little while. She said, "I don't feel like I can leave here today without telling you that your dad is showing all the signs of dying within one to two weeks." This was shocking.

We knew he was sleeping a lot. We knew he wasn't eating much or having bowel movements like he should be. We knew all these individual signs were present, but we were so close to it all, we couldn't see the whole picture. We were looking at each one as an individual problem. We figured we needed to take action on each of the individual challenges, such as increase his fiber or use medications to help move his bowels. In our minds, we needed to do all of these things to help my dad be able to continue to recover.

The truth was right there in front of us, and we just didn't see it—or didn't want to see it. Between the peace I had seen settle over him that morning, my answer from God, and the nurse's assessment, I knew it was time for me to be done fighting. It's a really tough thing to do when we want more than anything else for your loved one to stay with you.

It took some conversation and a little time for my sister to get there because she had not noticed the peace that I saw in him. We researched and had a conversation about bringing hospice in, and the next day we did just that. My sister struggled with this choice because hospice is a turn in the road. It's reaching a place where you either continue where you're going, which is to recover and return to health through medications, therapies, or whatever it takes to get there. Or you let go of those things, and you embrace allowing them to spend the time they have left controlling pain, helping with overall comfort, and getting the help that you need to be ready to let them go and for them to go.

There is confusion around hospice for many people. It's not only about dying. The services it provides can go on for a long period of time. They include health aides, RN visits, a social worker, as well as a chaplain. At the point they enter the picture, some medications are stopped and things like physical therapy are discontinued, depending on your loved ones needs.

We brought in hospice late Friday afternoon, and Dad passed away early Monday morning. It was a short period of time for our family to adjust to the thought of losing Dad. You can call and talk to hospice at any point if you're concerned about one of your parents and how they're doing. You will need a doctor's order for hospice to provide services, but an initial conversation with their staff can be helpful. One of the things I think hospice does well is share information on the signs to look for when the end of a life is near. They are able to give you an idea of what to expect along the road. That information is invaluable.

Dear Resistant Daughter/Son,

Life is full of change. You can embrace change for the benefit of you and your parent.

Your heart will break seeing the changes in your parent, and theirs will break, too, but your love and support will make a difference.

Keep focusing on this moment and the wonderful smile, laugh, or hug of today. You will survive the changes! Different doesn't have to be bad; it can be better.

Rayna

CHAPTER 6

Change Is Coming

I don't think anybody really loves change. There are some people who love the excitement of new things, but change for most of us is hard. It usually comes as a surprise. After we lost my mom, my dad was playing softball, traveling the country, and playing in tournaments. He also became a grandpa and enjoyed as much of his later years as he could without my mom. He and I also bought a business and were working together remotely.

One day, I was sitting in my office, and he called me. I asked, "What's up, Dad?" He told me he was worried about his memory. I said, "Oh, Dad, it's fine. I don't think you have anything to worry about. Why are you worried?" He let me know he just didn't seem to be remembering things like he used to. I said, "Yeah, but you're seventy-two years old, and you used to be younger. You know, we just don't really know what normal aging looks like." And he laughed.

My mom passed away at sixty-five, and my dad lost both of his parents before they were sixty. My mom's mom passed away at forty-three, and her dad was gone in his sixties. Our family didn't really know what normal aging was like. I told him to go to his doctor and tell him about his fears. I wanted him to do this to put his mind at ease, but I wasn't worried. He thought it was a good idea, and I thought that would be the end of it.

And it was the end of it until the day he called and asked when I was coming home next. I let him know I could come the following weekend but asked what was happening. He said, "We need to talk about what's going on because the results came back, and my memory is not what it should be." My heart sank. He said, "They're not saying Alzheimer's right now, but there is a problem, so we have some things to talk about."

The changes were right there on my doorstep, and I was not expecting this at all.

I think it's natural for us to be unwilling to accept change, even when it's right there in front of us. And it's harder if you're a fighter like me who wants to do everything possible to stop it. I think it's important for us to understand that what we struggle with about change is that our heads and our hearts aren't always on the same page. We have to view it as a challenge—how to get our head and our heart to the same place.

Sometimes, we don't believe the changes because we can't see them. Our mind isn't *getting it*. But oftentimes, our heart is what's really dragging behind with accepting the changes. The solution is that we can't ignore the changes. Ignoring them won't stop them. Life's going to go on. The difficulty is going to come, and we're going to have to learn how to live with it.

Manage Expectations

Looking at the changes and understanding what's truly changing is the first step. Acknowledging change is not easy. Having my dad diagnosed with the same disease that my mom died from was devastating. We knew what was coming. I knew that my dad wasn't going to know who I was by the time he passed away, and there's nothing easy about that.

Take the time to dig into the pain and find out why certain thoughts are coming to the forefront of your mind. What is it that's really pushing your resistance? Sometimes, it's simply that Dad's sick. It's the diagnosis that's devastating. But usually, it's deeper than that. There were many things that bothered me. *I live so far away; how am I going to be there for him. I can't imagine caring for him like I did Mom.* Wrestling with these thoughts, I realized it wasn't just that this was an Alzheimer's diagnosis; it was what was coming—watching my dad disappear before my eyes, like my mom did. *He will forget me like she did.* That hurt. That's what hung me up on not wanting to be willing to accept it or see it. Once I realized that future was what I was dreading, once I named it, even knowing I couldn't change it, it seemed to help me accept it in both head and heart.

At that point, I had to manage expectations. I knew I didn't want to have regrets. I didn't want to have *shoulds* and *woulds* and *coulds* and *I might have,* or *I would have,* or *it would have been better ifs.* Those things were not going to help me.

I had to be able to handle my fears about the timing and what was true. I lived four hours away from my dad. That was a truth. I asked myself, "What can I do? How can I take advantage of this time? How can I embrace this season of our lives?" I had to acknowledge that it didn't feel fair, that it really was hard, and it was going to get harder.

Relying on the truth of the Word was very helpful for me. Hebrews 13:8 tells us, *"Jesus Christ is the same yesterday, today and forever,"* and that brings me comfort. Jesus is the only thing that is never going to change. He had been there for me through my mom's disease and death. He would be there this time, too. While all of life is full of inevitable changes, He remains the same. No, we shouldn't have to go through this, but this is what's happening. Realize that Jesus is here for any of us as we walk through this season.

If you don't know Jesus and what He has done for you, I would love for you to check out the resources section in the back of this book to learn more about how to find peace in life through peace with Him. He offers the same peace I have with Him to everyone.

We could all benefit from learning to step into these situations and look for the positives. Hard news can feel devastating and overwhelming, and it's hard to even think about the positive aspects. When we get past the pain of "why," that's when we can start to move again. For me, I kept thinking, " I just can't do this again. There's no way I can do this again." When I stepped into my faith and said, "Okay, Lord, this is where we're going, and I know You're here with me," I knew I could do this again.

The truth is I can do this, and I can do this without regret.

That became my goal—looking for the positives in the situation—and it allowed me to get the most from the relationship with my dad as I could in the time he had left. Thankfully, I had fourteen years to do just that. I went to Disney World with him, my sister, and her family. I attended his softball games. We played volleyball together anytime I could make it. We regularly went bowling as a family. I played Ping-Pong with him. These were just a few of the fun experiences we shared, and it felt good to make the most out of the rest of the moments we had. With change, you need to find that state of mind that allows you to realize that it doesn't matter how you feel about it, because it's going to happen no matter what.

How can you understand your feelings and still do the best you can with what you have?

Fearing what was going to happen to my dad or fearing what might happen to me was not an option. Neither of these fears would make life better. Often, when people learn that both of my parents have passed away after journeying with Alzheimer's, they ask things like "Have you had the test to check if you have the gene that shows you're going to have Alzheimer's?" They don't quite say it out loud, but they do with their questions—*The odds of you getting Alzheimer's are very high; how do you live with that?* It's true—I know that family history is a factor, but fearing my future is not going to change anything.

Fearing the uncertainty of life will rob you of everything. After all, a car could hit me tomorrow. None of us know what's going to happen in the next five minutes, let alone ten years down the road. Overthinking things will steal your joy in the moment. Fear is typically driven by a lie, a story you're telling yourself that is not truth. The fear of having Alzheimer's is there, but there's just as likely a chance that I won't have to deal with it, so I choose to focus on that and leave the rest to God.

Look for the Positives

It's important to remember that your parent is still the same person they were, but things around them are changing. Things in them are changing and things about them are changing. It's important to acknowledge that this layered change is happening. Sometimes, they want to just put their heads in the sand, acting like none of it is happening, but the truth is, *it is* happening.

So, first understand that what's happening is natural. It's going to happen to me. It's going to happen to you. It could happen naturally through aging; it could be because of a disease like Alzheimer's. But we're all going to get to a place that we become more dependent on others to help meet our needs than we are right now. It's called aging. It's not about changing our roles.

Remembering aging parents as the people they were or are or continue to be is important. I always told the caregivers as much as I could about my dad as they came in to meet him. "My mom and dad married at seventeen and eighteen years old. My dad played baseball for the Brooklyn Dodgers. He spent a short time in the army and then went through night school and got his accounting degree. He worked for Folgers Coffee for most of his career and retired as the Chief Financial Officer of the Folgers Coffee plant in Kansas City. My dad loves sports. He loves to have things in order, and he loves to be in control."

Dignity and respect will help them stay stronger longer.

Acknowledge who your parents are and who they've always been and remember the things about them that make them who they are. When I get old, I hope people remember I'm a fighter because I'm not going to lie down quietly. It's just who I am. As much as things are changing for you, you have to remember that everything is changing for them, as well. They have been able-bodied adults for a long time, and they're now reaching a place where they have to be willing to ask for and accept help. Most of us are not very good at that.

As I watched my dad's disease progress, keeping the role of him being dad in the forefront of my mind was one of the goals I had, especially as I continued to help him with the more intimate needs he had as he progressed in the disease. He wasn't a child who needed help. He was an adult who needed help, and from day to day, how much help he needed varied.

Needs Will Change

Asking him questions and seeing what he was willing to let me do to help him made a big difference. Taking deep breaths. Staying in the moment and reminding myself how much I loved him also helped me to be able to serve him well and help take care of his needs. I think you have to let them make as many decisions as possible for long as possible. Our parents are adults, and they can make decisions until they've reached a point in which they can't. Even with Alzheimer's, there were still decisions Dad could make.

What time he wanted to go to bed was still a decision he could make, and I let him. Not taking all of the decisions away from our parent is really important. The more conversations you have with them, the more comfortable they are to accept the help. Building the trust, showing that you're there to support them, and doing what they need helps them gradually hand things over.

We were really worried about how my mom would handle not driving as she reached a point where it wasn't safe for her to be behind the wheel. We found she was actually thankful somebody else was taking that responsibility. My dad took early retirement from his job to stay home with her so the transition to him driving them around happened naturally. Not to mention, she probably scared herself way more times than she told anybody!

In fact, I'm not sure there ever was a conversation about her not being allowed to drive anymore because we didn't take away the keys. Her not driving didn't mean she had to stay at home and never do anything she wanted to do. It meant that someone else stepped in and started driving her to the places she needed to go and wanted to go. Dad was that person initially, and then caregivers stepped into that position.

The same thing was true with my dad. Since he was an accountant, money was something he managed really well. He intentionally saved to take care of my mom and himself in their old age. When it reached the point when he was having trouble balancing his checkbook or remembering where he'd written checks, he opened the door to the conversation by asking my sister, "Can you take a look at the bank statements and make sure everything looks right? Here are my investment statements. I just want you to keep an eye on them. If you have questions, I want you to know where things are, what I'm paying, and what I'm doing." It was a way for him to include her in the beginning. The more she asked questions, the more she showed that she could be responsible with it.

When Dad reached the point where he felt uncomfortable handling the money, he said, "I think I want you to take care of the bills for me."

She said, "Okay. Done." I never imagined he would have given that up. Allowing him to turn that over to her a little bit at a time, while keeping his dignity and showing him we respected his wishes, helped him stay stronger longer and let him know he was going to be taken care of. He knew we were going to do all that we could to keep him as happy and healthy as possible.

How you treat them makes a big difference
in the way they move forward.

I talk to many women who are in this season of taking care of a loved one. Sometimes, they don't have a good relationship going in, and I know that has to be really hard. I'm thankful that our family did have good relationships at the start of all of this. I think because of the experience he had with Mom as her primary caregiver, it helped him to know what to expect.

The rest of the family members were just support "staff" when he asked for help with her, and he didn't ask a lot. Dad knew he was going to need more care further into the diagnosis. He did a great job of having difficult conversations with us, talking about things no one wants to talk about. The ability to treat our parents with respect and build relationships of trust definitely allows your parents to hand things off without being embarrassed or worried that you're not going to do it the way they would want it done.

You Will Change Too

With all of this change occurring relationally, realize that moving into this role is going to change you, too. The changes are dramatic. I had a full life as a part-time teacher. I was also in school, working on my life coach certification. I had adult children and a high school student at home. I had a husband and a small business. I had volunteered at church, teaching Financial Peace classes. I did a lot of things and lived with a full plate.

Taking care of my dad's needs started slowly. With his diagnosis, I traveled home to him once a month. I made the time in my calendar to go and spend time with my dad. I started with baby steps, knowing that he was going to need more as time went on. There are no ifs or buts about it, my life changed dramatically the day we sat down and decided he would stay in his home.

For him to stay home, I needed to leave my home three and half days a week to care for him at his home. Integrating that responsibility into my already busy life had to happen. You can't just pile it on top of everything else you have to take care of and expect that you will be fine. That's not going to work! Spending time integrating those needs into your life slowly (if you have that kind of time) will make a big difference. If you've had a good relationship with your parents, then they've likely been your biggest cheerleader. Now it's your turn to come alongside and be there for them.

This season will expose your true character.

I'd say I'm strong-willed. Honestly, I would say I was more of a control freak. It's definitely been something I've worked on over my lifetime. As a business owner, I learned I couldn't control everything. I had to let go and let God control it. I had to trust the people who worked for me. I definitely had times throughout my adulthood where I learned to let go more and more but becoming one of Dad's caregivers revealed I wasn't doing quite as well as I thought in this area.

Stepping into this role of needing to care for my dad and wanting him to be as happy and healthy as possible was hard. I wanted to make sure he was safe and that everything was as good as it could be for him, but of course, I could not control everything. I found that my character quality of controlling things was helpful as long as I wasn't being over the top with it.

Becoming aware of his triggers really came in handy for me. When my dad put his baseball cap on, he was going somewhere. That was great when we were trying to get out the door, but not such a good idea at eleven o'clock at night. So the baseball cap had a place it stayed that was out of sight. It came out only when it was time to leave. Just learning how to control some of those things in his environment made things much easier. We didn't have to battle over him thinking it was time to go somewhere when it wasn't.

It also helped with unnecessary stressors. I wanted him to go to bed at a certain time because he had to wake up at a specific time to get to the day-stay facility, but he was eighty-four years old, and it was his choice. Letting go of those things and allowing him to make choices, continuing to offer him some other options, really helped me to understand that being a person who can control an environment can have its positives, but it also means that I can't govern it all the time. And again, I had to build trust in my faith, and I had to be willing to do what I could and let go of what I couldn't.

These changes help you boil down what is truly important. And ultimately, our most important things are being able to savor the relationships and enjoy that person we love so much and not let the little things, like getting out the door late, become big arguments. It's better to get out the door by joking around, sharing a smile, and building a memory, things that wouldn't have been possible if I had been stressed out and frustrated all the time.

It brought out in me the desire to be his voice and a voice to the world about this season. Talking about caregiving and end of life things is not what I would have ever thought I'd have a desire to do. They're not comfortable topics to talk about. They're hard and none of us want to sign up voluntarily, but I know that the experience we had with my dad will help others, and that is really important for me—helping others through this season so they can look back and not regret the things they did or didn't do.

It also helped me realize I'm only human. Sometimes, we think we can do more than we can. Watching our parents change and eventually walking them home hurts. That's just the way it is. My dad was a strong, smart, compassionate, loving dad who did amazing things. I can't say enough about who he was as a person. I wanted to be able to serve him without it hurting me so much, to be honest with you. Through that season, I wanted not to feel all those losses, but I eventually stopped pushing against them and started embracing the fact that it does hurt. We don't ever want our parents to leave. That's true, but it's part of the change.

Because I was just sixteen when my mom was diagnosed with Alzheimer's, in the process of losing her I thought, "If I stop caring and shut out the pain, it'll all be okay." Even as a teenager, I realized that really didn't help. Eventually, I broke down, and it was overwhelming. I learned to talk to the Lord through the daily difficulties of her not knowing where I was and her accusing me of not telling her where I was going and other hurtful experiences that happened.

I talked to the Lord through those things, so I could also experience all the things—the highs and the lows—and be able to take both the joy and the pain because that's the truth. Life is joy and pain. It's not one or the other. It's both.

Opening our hearts allows us to experience both joy and pain.

Through the sorrow and pain of watching my dad struggle with confusion and frustration, I learned to stop in that moment and acknowledge it—not ignore it or hold it in. Honestly acknowledging that these changes hurt and this season is hard made it where it didn't overwhelm me. I never stopped feeling like I wish it wasn't happening, but I also knew that wasn't something that could change. It was what it was. I needed to be able to share it with someone or be able to take it to God and ask Him to carry it with me.

Turning off our hearts to avoid experiencing the pain is not an option. Realize that God doesn't take it all away because we are human; we are going to have to deal with the pain. He helps us be in the moment and enjoy what we have right there. John 16:33 says, "I have told you these things, so that in Me you may have peace. In this world you will have trouble. But take heart! I have overcome the world." It's only with Him that I could find that peace during the very difficult times and have the hope that He gives us in that *take heart* part.

Notes

Dear Discouraged Daughter/Son,

Never forget! The heartbreak of the changes might cause you to forget who your parent is. Don't let it.

Though they are not who they once were, they are still who you have loved your whole life. They have taught you so much and shared their values with you, so honor them.

Spend time sharing memories with your parent; it will bring you both joy.

Rayna

CHAPTER 7

Remember Who They Are

This journey of taking care of a loved one is one that we'll all likely go through. We will have to jump into that role of caregiver and pick up where they no longer can. Throughout this book, I have talked about this topic, but I really feel it's worth investing an entire chapter on remembering whom your parent is. When we go through this season, we see our parent in a different light.

Being in this situation will change our perspective, but it's important, as we go through, not to ever lose sight of who they are, and the specialness of the person we're caring for. There is nothing more important than getting your mind wrapped around and holding on to that.

Embrace the Moment

Relationships change and people change. That's normal and natural, but in that parent-child relationship, we aren't often open to that change. We cling pretty hard to those roles we've always had before. Watching the changes in our parents is hard. But remembering who they are, not just in that moment and not just who they were in the past, but really just embracing the whole of our parents is such an important thing.

One of my sweetest memories with my dad in our caregiving season was playing Ping-Pong. I've talked about how much my dad loved sports. He loved to water ski and snow ski. He played handball. He played racquetball. He was an athlete, and a lot of his passions were wrapped around competition.

As we age, those things have to change and morph a little bit. With Alzheimer's, the ability to do those things he loved became more and more difficult. I mentioned he played volleyball with his senior friends; he did that multiple times a week up until three years before he passed. We had to stop that because his skin was getting so thin, and the ball caused injuries to his hands. This was very disappointing for him, but he was able to continue his gym workouts for an additional couple of years.

He loved being outside, but the summer heat in Missouri can be humid and brutal. As time when on, he wasn't able to handle that heat in the same way, so we had to adjust. After having a few scary situations with him being out in the sun, I had to look for ideas of how we could stay engaged physically and do those competitive kinds of things that he loved to do. I was at Walmart looking at the games, and I saw a Ping-Pong net, designed to go over a kitchen table. I picked that up and took it with me that next weekend. He had a formal dining room table we really didn't use, except to do puzzles. I put all the leaves in it, and I stretched that net across. I got the Ping-Pong paddles out, and I said, "Hey, Dad. Do you want to play?" A big smile came across his face—he loved that idea.

We played for nearly three hours that very first Saturday. I got my phone out and recorded some of those moments. We had so much fun. He was so ornery, cracked jokes, and we laughed, and it felt like I was a little girl playing with my daddy again. It is such a sweet memory. We played on that dining room table for a couple of weeks.

I came home after the second weekend and said to my husband, "Hey, we need a Ping-Pong table." He and I hit Craigslist, and I snagged one for seventy-five dollars and drug it up to Dad's house. We took over the formal family room as our official Ping-Pong room. That Ping-Pong table was there for years as we cared for Dad. It was a lot of fun for all of us—caregivers included. In fact, he played Ping-Pong just three days before we found the blood clot, which ended up leading to his death. Who would have ever thought that Ping-Pong could lead to such wonderful memories that allowed me to see the best in my dad?

Throughout all the changes, he could still hit the corner of the table and make me chase that Ping-Pong ball all the way down the hall, smiling at me as I ran. This was just one example of remembering who he was. Finding special moments that keep those parts of your loved one alive, active, and interactive helps you as well as them. When my dad hit that corner and the ball went flying down the hallway, it brought back that little girl moment of me playing with my dad.

Things like this allow us to embrace the person we love and remember him or her in a special way.

These are the memories that I have talked about and will continue to talk about as we move through this book. Being able to stay present with him and look for the smiles and the laughter and the ways to make him laugh made my day. There were times when he served three Ping-Pong balls at me at the same time, just because he was feeling ornery. It was awesome!

Honoring Your Parent

Remembering what your parents loved and did and incorporating those things into their current lives is something you can do, but it needs to be done intentionally. There are changes that will happen, especially with a horrible disease like Alzheimer's, things said, and behaviors observed that are just out of the norm—Dad said unkind things and sometimes hit, but it was important to remind myself that he was my dad, that he loved me and I loved him, and that I had to really pay attention to what honoring him would look like even in this season.

In the world today, we often honor esteem. We lift up famous people, such as movie stars, athletes, and people with power. Culturally, we have to stop and look at what honor looks like on an everyday basis because it is different for different people, but oftentimes, it's letting go of what used to be and embracing what is right there in the moment.

All relationships are going to grow and change. For me, the core value was honor. The Bible tells us, in Exodus 20:12, "Honor your father and your mother, so that you may live long in the land the Lord your God is giving you." This is a command that contains a promise. It's important for us to remember that we need to honor our parents, and if we do that, we're promised to have long life in the land that God has given us.

I found Dennis Rainey's book, *The Forgotten Commandment*, to have some interesting thoughts on this. The book is specifically about the commandment of honoring our parents. He recounts the time when he lost his dad suddenly to a heart attack. He said he was suddenly gone. There was no warning, no goodbyes. As Dennis stood by his dad's casket a few days after his death, regret filled his soul. He wanted to know why he hadn't expressed more of what he felt for his dad.

Many people find themselves in a place of regret when their parents are gone.

Dennis Rainey went on to say that he was able to find a way to go back and express that—to really visit the individual his dad was, to see him as a whole person, and go through a process of writing a tribute to his dad. This allowed him to not only be able to say the things he didn't say while his dad was here, but also Dennis made a pledge that he wouldn't wait until his mom was gone to come to grips with the impact that she had had on his life and ensure she knew how he really felt about her.

This book gives you an opportunity to walk through the process he walked through and be able to avoid having those regrets, learning how to express how you feel about your parents by honoring them with a tribute. Rainey also shared in his book about the promise that comes along with honoring your parents—you may live long in the land the Lord has given you.

God calls us to pass spiritual truth down from generation to generation, teaching our children in the way they should go, which, in turn, gives us multi-generational connections. The legacy of one generation is handed down to the next by honoring our parents.

Realize that when we really honor our parents, we do get to have those multiple generations of relationships, and we're able to see the things in our parents that we love and we want to pass on to our children, allowing that family legacy to move on. *The Forgotten Commandment* is a book I encourage you to take a look at and examine how you can give tribute to your parents while they're still here, or if you've lost them already, make that journey of walking through how to honor them even though they've passed.

In every situation, do your best to honor them in your speech.

Sometimes, we can let the way our parents talk to us impact how we talk to them. I found through my caregiving season that was the last thing I wanted to do. Sometimes it required taking a deep breath and walking away. For me, keeping my speech honoring and respectful to my dad was important.

There are five specific things that come to mind for me when it comes to remembering who your parents are:

- Honor their dignity.
- Respect their world.

- Consider their age.
- Discover what brings them joy.
- Provide for their basic needs.

Throughout this book, I have brought (and will continue to bring) all of these up, but I do want to briefly hit the high points of each one. Dignity is the right for a person to be valued and respected for his own sake. According to Wikipedia, *it's to be treated ethically*, and that goes back to the value and respect I have already talked about. This is not about what they can do for you or because of how they behave. There's no *if* in that. It's about honor and respect because that's what they deserve as a person. How we talk to an older adult or even a child changes how they talk to us.

Then it's about respecting their world. It's probably been a long time since you have lived with your parent, as most of us are adults. At this point, your worlds *are* very different. Generations are diverse. Their world is important to them, as is yours to you. Their routine and their preferences are their very own and may not align with yours.

My mom married very young and she wanted to be a mom more than anything else, but she didn't get pregnant until she was thirty-six years old. Before that she was a pharmaceutical buyer but as soon as she became a mom, she wanted to be at home. She was a homemaker who loved to read, bowl, and golf. She had a small group of friends; she had a beautiful smile. Mom loved to laugh, and she liked television comedies. She loved to listen to music.

Even after she changed because of Alzheimer's, we talked about the things that she had always been because those things were still true about her. She loved music and liked being at home and wanted to take care of people until the end of her life. We honored Mom by sitting with her and her dog listening to Elvis for hours and offering her the quiet peaceful environment she needed.

When it came to my dad, he had always eaten specific foods in certain ways, and that made him happy. It wasn't the same food I ate for dinner when I had a choice of what to make. But honoring him by doing what he would have done for himself if he could have was an important piece of respecting his world.

It's a pretty natural thing to reach a point in which it's probably not safe for aging parents to drive anymore. Many times, adult children come in and just tell them it's not safe anymore and that they are going to take their car. The conversation ends. That breaks my heart. As an adult who's in the season of life with kids and careers and all these other things that make us feel important, we would never be okay with someone coming in and taking our transportation away from us.

We have to think about how that affects our parents and understand that just because they're not able to drive anymore doesn't mean that they have to stay home and do nothing. For them to live a long and fulfilling life, we don't want them to do that. We have to find options to keep them active and able to get out and about. Respecting our parents' options to continue their regular lives and stay engaged in the world is definitely an important way of honoring them.

Next, we have to consider their age. Don't devalue them just because they can't do the things they used to be able to do. Limitations are expected. It's normal as time goes on that we can't do the same things we used to be able to do and being able to support them in the things they can do is important. Find ways to support, whether it be finding someone to do it for them or stepping in and taking care of things yourself.

Age doesn't make them any less of a person than they've been before.

Discover what brings them joy. Sometimes the really simple things can bring them joy. Think about what brings you joy. For me, it's a grandchild's smile or a husband's hug. Those things are simple. Our parents need those same simple moments of joy. You can start this long before you become a primary caregiver. Make that phone call once a week, have a monthly lunch date, meet them at church and take them to dinner afterwards. Of course, you may only be able to do the first one if distance separates you, but the point is to find the things that bring them joy. That is honoring them.

You really need to think about how you might need to step in to help provide for their basic needs. Aging is expensive. Hopefully your parents have planned ahead, and money is not a concern for them, but for a lot of people, that's not the reality. I'd like to challenge you to ask if money is a concern for your parents. Our parents don't usually want to talk to us about their money, but the last years of their lives are the most expensive. Typically, this is because of medical expenses. Seventy-five percent of people die in the hospital or a nursing home, so the death of a parent can significantly impact the reserves they had for the surviving parent.

Plan When Possible

My mom died twenty years before my dad did. The amount of investment it took to take care of her while she was living through her twelve-year journey through Alzheimer's was quite substantial, but that was something my dad knew he wanted to take care of. I don't think he ever imagined he would live twenty years longer than her.

I'm so thankful that he had planned ahead because we were able to provide for him, to step in and give him the kind of care that he wanted, with what he had saved. But many times, parents haven't saved enough, and they're not able to provide for their retirement in the same way they expected, especially if medical illnesses are a reoccurring theme in their marriage or lifetimes.

Stepping in and helping your parents when their money might be tight is helpful. You might be surprised what they're doing to make ends meet. Many seniors are skipping meals or even discontinuing medication because they find they don't have the financial resources they need. It's important to know where they are and if their basic needs are being met.

When the time comes, I won't want to ask my kids for help. I think that's normal. We raised them; we took care of them. Kids are the last people our parents want to admit to that they're struggling. Honestly, this is a conversation you need to be having even before you are technically caregiving. If you can help them make some decisions or understand something better early on, it might avoid an issue in the years to come.

When my father-in-law passed away, there were a lot of details with the farm that my mother-in-law had to step in and take care of, and it could have been overwhelming for her. Having the support of the kids to answer those questions and check in to see she's doing okay made a huge difference.

Dear Honoring Daughter/Son,

Don't be fooled by the increased needs of your parent. They are still the same people who have loved you since you were conceived, making every sacrifice they could raising you.

Stay on the lookout for your "all or nothing" thinking. The answers that honor everyone are often found somewhere in the middle ground. Asking questions is the quickest way to find the initially unseen options.

You are doing a good job of staying in the moment; it really is where the joy is found.

Rayna

CHAPTER 8

Navigating Balance

I n the last chapter, we talked about remembering who your parent is, but I wanted to take some time to dive deep into the fact that you really must remember that your parent is an adult. They've made their own decisions for a very long time, and now for the first time, they are forced to rely on help from others. When stepping in to help, you're stepping into a very sensitive area for them.

There's no way to put this softly; this is one of the hardest things they will ever have to do. They are giving up their independence, and it's you, their child, stepping in to help them. You need to appreciate that they are still a grown person. They do still have an opinion, and they do have a right to that opinion.

Staying in the Moment

I think asking questions is a big key to navigating this part of the journey successfully. It's funny how we, as humans, are oftentimes all in or have nothing to offer. We want to come in and take over everything, or we want to be completely hands off. Finding that balance as we're navigating the aging process with our parents is so important. It's okay to walk beside them and simply acknowledge that things are getting hard, and it's okay to ask questions if you do it carefully. Navigating with questions allows them to hear you and not think you're trying to control them completely.

One example of how you might navigate this is on a hot summer day ask, "So, how's your lawn mower working? It's pretty hot this summer. What if I came over and ran the lawn mower and you weed eat?" Your goal is to ask in ways they can openly accept the help, but you need to realize that if they tell you no, it's no for now. You can always revisit the question later. It's important to come from a place of caring when they're in need.

Staying in the moment with a parent emotionally can make a big difference.

Things will change over the time you are taking care of a parent. There will be times you will have to remember that you love them. I had a really difficult time with my dad some nights. I put him to bed three nights a week, and there was never any consistency to when he would get frustrated with me. The main issue that would come up was getting him to take off his pants.

Being able to allow him to have his dignity and accomplish what needed to be done meant that I needed him to change into his pajamas. Toward the end of his life, we were dealing with more incontinence—during the day as well as at night—and he had a special brief that he needed to wear at night.

I still let him choose what time he wanted to go to bed, but I had to be sure that he changed into his pajamas. I would walk with him to his room and show him where his jammies were and ask him to go ahead and take off his clothes and get ready for bed. Two nights out of three, it would be a ten-minute process, no big deal. That one night when it was a big deal was difficult. At times there was even some name calling and hitting.

He had a small bathroom off of his bedroom, and I could ask him to go change in there on these challenging nights. That way, I could stand in the doorway and physically keep him in the bathroom until he changed his clothes.

Typically, he wouldn't try to get by me. It would just be me standing there, asking him over and over; "Dad, can you take off those pants and put these on, please? . . . Dad, can you take off those pants and put these on? . . . Dad, can you take off those pants and put these on?" That would normally work pretty well, but some nights, it could last an hour and a half. Sometimes, he would say yes, and then not do it. Obviously, on the nights that it took that hour and a half, the frustration would be building and building for both of us.

I was always looking for ways to try to stay honoring in what I was saying to him, give him his dignity, and still accomplish what needed to be done. One weekend, after a very rough Saturday night, I came home on Sunday, and I was telling my husband about how hard it was. He said to me, "Rayna, what would happen if you were to just hug your dad and tell him that you loved him?"

I explained that he would likely hit me. I was taken aback that he would even ask me that, and I felt like he just didn't understand. I assumed he had no idea what he was talking about or how I felt. I blew him off, and we went about our day. I went to see Dad the next weekend, and there I was in the bathroom doorway again.

"Dad, can you take off your pants and put these on?" He was not going to have it, and he was getting more and more frustrated with me. On this night, he wanted to get out of the bathroom, past where I stood. He was saying, "Excuse me!" I stayed calm and told him, "I'm sorry, I need you to put these clothes on before we can go back in the bedroom." He was getting really upset with me.

I remembered what my husband said, and I thought, "Well, I'll just give it a try." I wrapped my arms around him; he stiffened up and his fists were clenched. He stood there stiff as a board as I wrapped my arms around him, and I started patting him on the back. I said, "Daddy, I love you. You're okay."

I held him. I kind of rocked him a little bit and patted him on the back and just kept repeating that statement in different ways, "Daddy, I love you. I'm here to help you. You're okay." I held him until he relaxed into my hug. Eventually, he laid his head on my shoulder, and he let me hold him. I continued to tell him I loved him and that he was okay.

I held him for a while and eventually I dropped my arms, and I stepped back a little bit. He looked me in the eyes, and he said, "What do you need me to do?"

I said, "Daddy can you just take off your pants?"

That sounds like a funny thing to say in the moment, but he said, "Sure," and he did. He changed his pants and went to bed. I remembered that night from then on. I could give him a gentle pat and remind him who he was. *Daddy, I love you. You're okay, and I'm here to help you.* And he was able to respond (most of the time) and do what I asked him to do.

It didn't work one hundred percent of the time. It wasn't a magic wand experience, but it was a moment each time that gave him the reassurance that I was there to help. And with honor and respect, I was able to accomplish what I needed to accomplish to safely get him tucked in at night., giving him a kiss goodnight and leaving him there to rest for the evening.

Honoring Their Passions

Interacting in that caring way can bring some remembrance and calm to those tough moments. In a situation like this, it's easy to allow ourselves to get out of control, which can cause turmoil. By navigating the balance of where you are right at that second will allow you stay in the moment. I had to remember to be playful with my dad because that is who he was. He enjoyed being playful. Our family room, kitchen, formal dining, and formal living room were all in a circle around the stairs that went downstairs and upstairs on the main floor. Sometimes I'd be looking for him and calling for him, and I couldn't find him anywhere. Then I'd see him peeking around the corner; he was playing hide-and-go-seek with me, just grinning up a storm. I had to remember not to get frustrated in that moment but instead laugh with him. It allowed me to have fun with my dad. That's very important.

Remember that letting them be who they are lets you be who you are, as well.

In Chapter Three, I talked about what brings a parent joy. Sometimes, we get in the mentality of being focused on the work to be done and we forget about the emotional state of whom it is we're doing that work for. This goes back to remembering who they are and what they love. When we're adults, we may not even remember what our parents love because we have been involved in our own lives for so long. While we come together as a family to celebrate things, we don't necessarily engage in their everyday life after we are adults.

What did they do when they had a choice? It might be playing cards; it might be bowling; it might be golfing; it might be going to church or attending daily mass. There are lots of things that our parents did when they were independent. How did they spend their free time when they had it? If you can keep them involved in those things as long as possible, you're going to help them remain in a place of delight. They're going to experience the joy of life. They're going to experience purpose, and that's important at all stages.

Finding those activities makes such a big difference. As I mentioned earlier, my dad was an athlete, and because he was an accountant by trade, he was extremely driven by problem solving. He was a thinker, but he loved sports, and keeping himself physically active was the joy of his life.

In thinking about my mom, she was a whole different person. When I think about the mom I remember, she enjoyed bowling, golfing, crocheting, watching a movie, and she was always reading a good book. She was professional before she had children, but once we came along, she loved being a homemaker and mom. She volunteered at the elementary school library and was the classic PTA mom.

All of those things about her were important to consider as we cared for her. It was harder for me because I was just a teenager when she was diagnosed, so this season of caring for my mom was different. I didn't know as much about how to help her as I did with my dad. I do remember that she would get restless, so I would take the tea towels out of the drawer and make a big pile on the table. "Hey, mom, can you help me fold these?" We folded the towels, and she'd make a nice stack, and then I would throw them back on the table again to start over.

This activity kept Mom with me, in the moment, and was a time of joy for both of us.

For years after her diagnosis, my mom dried the dishes. When my dad took over cooking, he didn't like to use a dishwasher, so he washed the dishes by hand, and Mom was the official dryer. For a long time, Mom could put those dishes away on her own, and then she got to a place where she couldn't find where the dishes went. She progressed to a place where she was dropping things and breaking them, but we found new ways to allow her to dry. Even if it was a Tupperware bowl that wasn't even dirty, we let her dry the plastic items so that she could do things that gave her joy. She loved to help and being a part of what was going on around her.

Mom also loved music. Elvis and Nat King Cole were her favorites; she spent hours in that formal family room listening to records and singing along. As her disease progressed, her words weren't really words but melodies that she made by clapping her hands with the songs. That was one of the things that she spent hours doing with her little dog by her side.

Finding ways to bring your parents joy will keep them happier and with you longer. It's really just a matter of stepping back and thinking about the things you already know about them and then figuring out how you can adapt those things to allow them to continue to engage as long as possible.

These are the kinds of things that would be easy to miss if you don't know what to expect.

It can be easy to allow ourselves to get caught up in a situation and to think more about what we have to do than the person we are doing it for. This puts the focus on us, and we can lose the focus we need to have on them. Remember this season is hard on them—likely the hardest time of their lives. As caregivers, we want this time to be as easy as possible for them, not for us. So take the time to really dive deep into what your parents love and what makes them happy, and then find creative ways to integrate those activities into your day to make their journeys as comfortable as you can. If you remember they are adults and treat them as such, bringing joy to their lives, you'll find that in the end, you'll have moments to reflect on that will give you peace and comfort and less regrets.

Dear Caring Daughter/ Son,

You are doing a wonderful job caring for your parent.

What caring looks like will change throughout your journey. Keep on the lookout for the best way to meet the needs of your parents and yourself.

Checking in during a quiet moment can help you see what you need or what your parent needs during this season, and remember to do this often.

Everyone knows how much you care; it's okay to not do it alone.

Rayna

CHAPTER 9

Getting the Best Care Possible

There was a time in both my mom and dad's journeys that we knew we needed help. It's not really a question of if you will need outside help during your season of caring; it's more of a question of when you need help and how to make sure you're getting the best help you can get.

My mom's diagnosis came as I was beginning my junior year of high school, so I had a couple more years at home, but then I went off to college. I was gone from home just a year when my dad decided to take early retirement and be home with my mom full time. He did it for a couple of reasons. One, he was definitely concerned that her disease had progressed, and he was uncomfortable with her being home alone all day. Two, he wanted to be able to do as much with her as he could. They were in their early fifties and had wonderful plans for retirement, plans that were cut short.

Dad played softball three times a week, plus had practices. He started out taking Mom to his softball games, but it got to a point where going to softball practice and all of the games became too much for my mom. She would get up and wander a little bit during games, which made it difficult for him to focus.

They also had plans to travel, but with her decreasing abilities, he knew it wouldn't be long before that wasn't possible. It was "now or never" for spending as much time together as possible.

Everyone Needs Help

I was living in Texas during the middle part of my mom's illness. It was a nine-hour drive, much too far away from my parents. It was at that time when my dad decided he needed some help. I remember being impressed that he was willing to ask for help.

I would go up and visit as much as I could, but it was not often enough to give my dad all the help he needed. My best friend in college, Monica, moved up to the area where my parents lived, and Dad asked if she would be interested in staying with my mom a couple days a week. That's the first step my dad took in getting help for taking care of my mom.

Monica had a little girl, and they would go and spend the day with my mom. This made it possible for my dad to get out and go to softball practice, get to the gym, and do the grocery shopping—things that had become a struggle with mom at that point. He was quick to let go of the housekeeping, too, so Monica vacuumed and dusted. Mom was able to help her with that, which she loved.

This gave Mom someone else to spend time with, someone who also ensured she was safe. That was a really good fit for a period of time. Monica had another baby, so she wasn't available to help any longer. Dad found someone else, and he increased the amount of time the caregiver was there. Eventually, he had help five days a week for eight hours each day.

Knowing that mom was safe at home allowed him to get out and engage with people and do things he liked to do. He volunteered to do taxes for seniors, run errands, and continue all the hobbies he liked to do. He was never willing to turn everything over to someone. For instance, he didn't let anybody get Mom up in the morning or bathe her. He kept those things for himself. Sometimes, I would send him away when I came home for Spring Break, or over the summer when I was teaching, or my sister would help care for her when he had an out-of-town softball tournament, but most of the time, most of the caregiving tasks fell on his shoulders. Eventually, I moved back to the area and was able to take over some evenings and Saturdays while he was playing softball.

Asking for help was difficult for Dad, and accepting it was also a challenge. He felt like he needed to do it all. All of us can feel that way, but it's important to understand that asking for help is not admitting a weakness but rather showing strength. Recognizing that you can't do it all and humbling yourself enough to admit you need help will get you to the help you need much faster and easier.

Later, as I was in that role of helping to care for Dad, I knew I needed help. Even though we had set the team up properly in the beginning, there were times when things would change with his patterns or his behaviors over the four-and-a-half-year period.

I had to routinely look at what was working and what was not working.

There was a season when he was not sleeping well. He would get up four to five times a night. With me being there three nights in a row, it was difficult having my sleep interrupted like that. I'm a sleeper, and I know I need my sleep. I mentioned to my sister that things were not going well, and I thought I needed the morning caregiver to stay a little bit longer for me to be able to get the sleep I needed to be available for him at night.

Making adjustments to the schedule was a bit simpler because we had those conversations. We were able to look at what was working and what wasn't working well so that we could ask for help. Still, that's not an easy thing to do. It's important to talk about this from the beginning, as soon as you start noticing issues. If your family's goal is to keep your parents in their home as long as possible, then you're going to need help to do that. Just realizing that help is needed is a big first step.

If you have one parent who is in a role of taking care of the other parent, it's important to get help in there where you can, because this time of caregiving will have a significant impact on both of their health. The spouse who is in a caregiving role typically has a lot of medical issues once that other spouse passes because they usually neglect their own health.

Having the freedom like my dad did when he was taking care of my mom to go to his own doctor's appointments, to get the exercise he needed, and to get some relief from the constant responsibility of caregiving was imperative. Make sure you have conversations about the caregiver's health and how they need to be open to help as early as possible.

Take Inventory

Knowing when to bring in help for your parent can be challenging. Take an inventory of needs by asking questions. How are your parents doing? What tasks did the sick parent take care of that they're no longer able to handle? What tasks are they struggling with? How do they feel about tasks, such as taking care of the house and yard?

You have to ask on a regular basis, *how's it going?* Many of my clients notice a big change when one parent passes away. All of the responsibilities suddenly fall on one person, and it can be very over-whelming. Be sure to check in with your remaining parent. Ask what it was the parent who is gone used to do. Sometimes one parent does the bookkeeping and the other doesn't know a whole lot about the money. Or one parent handled the housework, and the other is not sure what to do when. Making sure they're comfortable with the things they aren't used to taking care of and offering to help or find help for them will usually be welcomed. You just have to ask to see where you can be of assistance.

That's one thing I learned from when my mom was sick. I was young, but I didn't think to ask my dad those questions to make sure that he was taking care of himself. I knew that he had brought help in, but I don't know if there was more that I could have done when I look back now.

Taking inventory of the needs also includes making sure the house is safe for your parent. As we age, our physical needs change. Are grab bars needed in the shower or by the stool? Is there enough light on the inside and the outside, along the walkways and driveways? Aging eyes don't work as well, and more light is required. Are there any big changes that need to be made to the home to make it safer?

Where is the laundry room? In my dad's home, the laundry was in the basement. My dad was physically able to go up and down those stairs for all of his life up until the very end, but my mom wasn't able to navigate the stairs. For many people, going up and down stairs is a big safety issue. If he wasn't able to navigate the stairs well, we would have had to consider either moving the laundry room or hiring help to take care of the laundry. The last thing you want is an accident on the stairs.

Are there certain things that they need help with as far as maintenance around the house such as painting the house or cleaning the windows? Think about all the things that they normally have taken care of on their own that now might not be safe for them to continue to do.

Taking an inventory is really important. Once you've looked at how they're doing and the things that might need to be addressed, it's time to have a conversation with them. Then, it's a matter of finding the best people to meet those needs. It might be you, it might be another family member, or you might need a professional.

If you look at that list and you choose to take on everything on it, you're overwhelming your own life, and that's not the best thing you can do for them. I encourage you to stop and consider what the best solution is once you know everything that they need help with. This list will be dynamic. As time goes on, they may need more help on one or more areas.

There is no one who can manage a home and take care of all the physical and emotional needs of someone else twenty-four seven and still live a viable life. If you're doing this alone, you're really doing everybody a disservice. Your parent wants and needs your help but not at the cost of your marriage, career, or mental health. Enlisting help will make a difference.

Notes

_____

_____

_____

_____

_____

_____

_____

_____

_____

_____

_____

_____

_____

_____

_____

_____

_____

_____

_____

_____

Dear Team Player,

You are an important part of the team. Being on a team requires patience, wisdom, and confidence in your role.

As a daughter/son, you will likely be managing all the players on your team—your parents, their doctors, the caregivers, and even the individual who mows the lawn.

You can be compassionate, supportive, and friendly while being clear about the needs and responsibilities with each team member. Communication will be the key to helping the team run smoothly.

Rayna

CHAPTER 10

It Takes A Team

D ad already had someone who was mowing the grass for him because that interfered with how often he got to play ball. But the longer he lived, the harder it became to stand inside the house watching someone else mow his grass. It really bothered him.

Finding chores he could do in the yard to help while the yard person was there was helpful. Dad loved to rake the leaves. He did not like leaves in his grass, and so he spent a lot of time taking care of removing leaves. It made him feel like he was taking care of things. Once it got to the point that he couldn't handle the whole yard, his job was to make sure the back deck was clear. Sometimes, I even sprinkled leaves on the deck just to give him a job and make it easy for him to participate. Allowing him to stay engaged and do what he was capable of doing as long as he could brought him joy.

It takes a team, and you do have to
bring in people to support you.

Caring for their personal needs will change over time. When Dad developed melanoma and had surgery to have the skin cancer removed, it was a rough situation for all of us. He had quite a long journey back to physical health after that surgery. His personal needs became something he couldn't take care of on his own at that time. My dad showered and shaved every morning, every day. While not everybody wants to do that, that was who Dad was.

We wanted to continue to allow him to do that, so we brought caregivers in. From the time of his release from the hospital to the end of our caring season, we had caregivers that came in and bathed and assisted him as he shaved every day so that he could maintain his lifestyle the way he would have if he could.

Dad started his day with a caregiver every morning, waking him up at the same time and helping him with his morning routine habits. His days were spent at the day-stay facility or with a caregiver, and then a family member came in and filled in from there and on into the nighttime routine. Those were the types of things that we saw he needed help with, so we just started stepping into those roles or finding someone to fill those duties, as he needed it.

It is okay not to have to do it all yourself. Anybody who's worked with a team to take care of a loved one knows that a team is not always comprised of family members or people who know your parent. As you put that team together and as you get outside people involved, it's important that you get them on board with the mission.

Routine Helped Dad

One of the most important things to keep in mind is that folks care more and do more for the people they care about. Part of our process was to be very specific in what we were asking for as we hired caregiving help. Not everyone is like my dad; he was a very routine-oriented person.

I would explain to the caregivers that were caring for him about my dad's life and how he had taken that exact brown paper sack lunch to work every day. He ate the same thing for lunch every day. That tells you a lot about who he is. Routine was extremely important to him. Right after his surgery, when he wasn't able to do things for himself, we sat and wrote down exactly how he got ready in the morning.

What did he do first? Did he get in the shower first, or did he brush his teeth first? When he was in the shower, did he wash his hair first, or did he wash his body first? We went through every detail of his bathing routine. With that information, we were able to ensure that he was able to continue to do what he wanted to do every day.

We provided the support that it took for him to do that by creating a checklist of each of his routines. Every person who came in to care for my dad was trained in his routine. I emphasized over and over again, that this is what he would do if he could do it himself, and our goal was to help him be able to continue it.

No matter who was helping him, it needed to always look the same.

We made sure they understood how important routine was for him. Our goal was for them to support him and reduce his frustration, not to do it for him. It's not respectful to do something for somebody if they can do it for themselves. Though he had a disease that sometimes caused him not to be able to do things, for the most part, all the way up until four weeks before he passed, he could brush his teeth, he could get in the shower, and he bathed himself and dried himself off.

Some days, the caregiver might have to put the toothpaste on the toothbrush, hand it to him, and he would go right for it and start brushing his teeth. There were other days where he might look at that toothbrush and not know what to do with it. They might have had to move it to his mouth and start moving it up and down, but then he would take over. Each day was a little different. Our encouragement to his caregivers was to let him do as much for himself as he could.

He could always dry himself. Of course, sometimes they had to help him dry the middle of his back, but to dry him when he was capable of doing that after getting out of the shower would have been extremely uncomfortable for him. We made sure the entire caregiving team understood those expectations. We also made sure they understood our family dynamic.

We showed them family pictures. We talked about my mom, especially because she wasn't there anymore. There were pictures of her in his bedroom; we would talk about who she was and how long she had been gone and the sacrifices that my dad made to take care of her so the team understood who he was as a man. We talked about all parts of his life. We talked about sports and the things he loved to do in his spare time. We walked each person who came into our home through an introduction of our home, our family, and our goals and mission of keeping him home as long as possible. We recruited them to be a part of that.

Effective Communication

We wanted the outside caregivers to understand why routine was so important. We wanted them to fall in love with my dad. Many of the caregivers that took care of my dad grieved him almost as much as they would have a family member when he was gone because we really did embrace them and ask them to be a part of our family.

You want the caregiving team members to buy in and give you their best efforts in supporting your loved one.

My dad taught me in business that communication is key. As we were in business together, he would remind me, "Have meetings, Rayna. Sit down and talk with people. Find out where they're coming from." That was definitely something we implemented with our caregiving team.

We had as many as twelve people managing my dad's care, being at home with him, and cleaning the house—all the different pieces that needed to be done—so it was really important that we talked. We had communication in writing, by utilizing checklists on the wall for everyone to see. We had checklists they filled out in notebooks to give us feedback. We passed information and questions back and forth.

- What time did he have breakfast?
- How much of his breakfast did he eat?
- Did he get his medication down?
- How much of his medication was taken?

Bob's Day

Day/Date: _Sunday_____

Morning Routine

Caregiver Name: _____

Shake: __ No __ Yes Time: ___ : ___ AM

What time did Bob get out of bed?

_____ : _____ AM

How easily did he get up?

1   2   3   4   5

Easily   Very Difficult

Wet

__ Brief   __ PJs   __ Pad

Pain Level

1   2   3   4   5

None   Very bad

Mood

1   2   3   4   5

Great   Not nice

Confusion

1   2   3   4   5

Very Clear   Very confused

BM   __ Yes   __ No

Bathroom

__ Shower   __ Partial Cleaned
__ Shave   __ Lotion
__ Teeth Brushed __ Other _____

Overall Comment – Morning Routine

_____
_____

Breakfast

Medication

1   2   3   4   5

No Problem   Did not get any in him

Medication comment

_____
_____

What was for breakfast?

__ Eggs   __ Juice
__ Cereal   __ Waffles
__ Oatmeal   __ Sausage
__ Toast   __ Fruit/Banana
__ Other_____

How much did he eat?

__ 100%   __ 60%
__ 90%   __ 50%
__ 80%   __ Less than 50%
__ 70%   __ Other _____

Breakfast comment _____

_____

Blood Pressure – Time Taken

_____ : _____ AM

Blood Pressure & Heart Rate – Readings

_____ / _____   _____

Weight _____

Trash ___ Yes   ___ No

Laundry ___ Yes   ___ No

Overall morning comment

_____
_____

Daytime

Where did Bob spend the day?

__ Home   __ Shalom Day Stay

AM Activity

__ At Shalom   __ Read books/paper
__ Ping pong   __ Sat outside
__ Puzzle   __ Other _____
__ Nap   _____

Lunch – Time (Note: Please leave blank when eating at Shalom)

_____ : _____ AM or PM

Lunch - Meal

__ At Shalom   __ Veggies
__ Ham sandwich   __ Water
__ Turkey sandwich __ Juice
__ Chips   __ Sprite
__ Other _____

How well did he eat lunch? (Note: Please leave blank when eating at Shalom)

1   2   3   4   5

All of it   None of it

Lunch comment _____

Afternoon Activity

__ At Shalom   __ Nap
__ Gym   __ Read books/paper
__ Ping Pong   __ Sat outside
__ Puzzle   __ Other_____

Caregiver Name: _____

2:00 Meds

__ At Shalom   __ Yes   __ No

BM   __ Yes   __ No

Evening

Caregiver Name: _____

What's for Dinner?

_____
_____

Dinner – Time (Note: Please leave blank when eating at Shalom)

_____ : _____ PM

How well did he eat dinner? (Note: Please leave blank when eating at Shalom)

1   2   3   4   5

All of it   None of it

Dinner comment _____

Time arrived home _____ : _____ PM

PM Activity

__ Help w/ Dishes   __ Read books/paper
__ Ping Pong   __ Sat outside
__ Puzzle   __ Other _____
__ Nap

Comment _____

Night Routine

Snack

__ Rice Dream   __ Cookie/Brownie
__ None   __ Other _____

Medication

1   2   3   4   5

No Problem   Did not get any in him

Medication comment

_____

Blood Pressure – Time Taken

_____ : _____ PM

Blood Pressure & Heart Rate – Readings

_____ / _____   _____

Mood

1   2   3   4   5

Great   Not nice

PJ's and white brief   __ Yes   __ No

Cream on left knee and lower back

__ Yes   __ No

BM   __ Yes   __ No

Time in Bed _____ : _____ PM

Overall evening comment

_____

Slept all night?   __ Yes   __ No
If No, woke up & out of bed at:

Time: _____ : _____ AM or PM
Time: _____ : _____ AM or PM
Time: _____ : _____ AM or PM

Other comments _____

All of that information not only helped my sister and I as we managed the situation, but also assisted caregiver-to-caregiver communication. My sister is a texter, and she routinely checked in with caregivers. "How is your day going? How is dad doing?" She had constant communication with them via text.

I was there in the home with them as they were caring for him much of the weekends, having conversations with them and asking each person who was leaving a shift to tell the person who was coming in how the day was going, what they had been doing, how much time he'd spent doing different activities, and to try to move him on to something else if they needed to.

Hiring caregivers is a challenge that can't be taken lightly.

There are hundreds of home care companies out there. One of the most important things to know when you make the phone call to interview a home care company is to understand that you're talking to a salesperson. There's nothing wrong with salespeople, but they're definitely selling you their services. They're going to put their best foot forward in the beginning when they handle your inquiry, get back to you or return your phone calls quickly, and send professional people to your home to assess whether they can provide the care for you.

As a person who's been in sales with my business before, I could see those things. My sister had been an accountant and then a stay-at-home mom, so she didn't always see the things I did. Whenever we were looking at hiring a new company, and they weren't keeping deadlines or returning phone calls, she would have an excuse for them.

I let her know that if they're doing this before being hired, it's going to be worse later because right now, they are fighting for our business. This is a business transaction, and it needs to be treated that way. They are our employees. It is important to get started in a very professional manner, laying out expectations and making sure you've been clear on exactly what you're looking for.

Like Family

Caregivers are going to be like a part of the family, but they're not family—you do have to keep that in mind. My sister and I also learned, because we had different strengths and different personalities, both of us needed to be a part of the hiring process. I usually did the initial screening, asked the initial questions, discussed our needs, laid out the expectations, and then set up a time for her to meet them face to face.

If we both weren't in agreement, we didn't go with that company or didn't allow that caregiver to work for us. Even when we were looking at day opportunities for Dad, we would go at various times to tour the facilities and see different people because we wanted to be sure that we were both being given consistent information.

When we came back and compared notes, it was interesting to see and learn what the other person experienced on the tour. It gave us the best information possible in the process of finding the right people to provide that care for my dad.

As I mentioned earlier, we did not allow anyone to take care of Dad until they had met my dad and at least one of us, and they had gone through our training. This happened while we were right there in the house with them; we introduced them to what was expected. We had to all agree if it would be a good fit or not. This is not normal for home care companies, but we felt it's necessary to be as thorough as possible to make sure to get the best help possible.

They typically want to send anyone who's available to cover that shift. That was not okay with us. We wanted Dad to like the person and know they would be able to interact well together. We could see those things in the process of the interview and training. We were up front with the companies about expecting our team of people to have all met my dad and have been through our instruction, and those were the only people we allowed to come into Dad's home.

If they had a problem covering a shift, they would have to call us and tell us they weren't sending anybody. It's not something they wanted to do as a business, but it did happen occasionally. When it started happening often, we knew it was time to start looking for a different company because it was only going to get worse.

I really feel introducing the caregiver to your loved one and the family is imperative. Explaining the challenges of the situation brought understanding. The fact that I was driving two hundred and twenty miles one way to be a caregiver for my dad helped the caregivers understand the sacrifices that our family was willing to make to be sure he had the best care possible.

Meeting Aunt Colleen, Robin, and me was important for them to understand what our mission was and to invite them to be a part of that, to really see they were going to be part of this team that was focused on making my dad's life as good as possible.

We all do more than what's expected
for people we care for. We just do.

We get up at the crack of dawn to take the people we care about to the airport, or we wake up in the middle of the night to help change a tire for them. We do whatever it takes for those we love. We wanted the caregivers to see that this was not just a job, but it truly was about being a part of our family and joining us with helping my dad the best way that we can as a team.

It was not unusual for us to ask them, "How are you doing? What can we do differently? What will make your job easier?" We had specific expectations so that if something wasn't getting done, we had conversations about it.

Most of the caregiving companies said they would do light housework. There was no one was living in the home twenty-four seven, except my dad. The rest of us were coming and going, so it was really important that light housework was done regularly or the house became filthy. Even those responsibilities were on our checklist, so it was easy to notice what wasn't always getting done.

We would have "check-in" conversations with the caregivers that gave us the opportunity to ask about things like the living room not getting vacuumed or bathrooms not being cleaned. At one point, we were hearing they didn't have time. Sometimes, it didn't feel like it was the truth, but who's to say? Since it wasn't happening, we stepped back and decided to re-evaluate.

We chose to cut back their time by half an hour and pay someone to specifically come and clean the house every week. That way we knew that piece of the caregiving was done regularly. Making an adjustment like that was something we did often. We'd check in and keep an eye on how things were going and adjust where necessary.

While we did have to keep in mind that the caregivers were there because they were being paid to be there, we wanted to make sure they knew how much we appreciated what they were doing, too. We gave them Christmas gifts. We sent thank you cards and gave occasional gift cards to Starbucks and places like that when they went above and beyond their duties. Some caregivers even brought gifts on Dad's birthday. We wanted them to know how much it meant to us that they really cared and loved him. Robin and I valued and appreciated those who cared for him.

We found a good balance between high expectations and tangible acts of appreciation.

If you can make people feel like what they're doing is part of their purpose, not just something they have to do, they will certainly do a better job, which will bring a better result. While they know it's a job, you are making them feel part of the bigger picture. Just like with all teams, there were times we decided we couldn't move forward with a team member or it might be time to refresh the team.

Over this four-and-a-half-year period, we fired four home-care companies. It was never a permanent relationship. We wished it could have been, but it seemed like we would start out strong, and eventually, we would be moved lower and lower on their priority list. At least, that's how it felt from our family's perspective. While I think it's valuable to treat them like family, you also have to remember they're employees. We did have to draw that line and make it clear that there was an expectation that the job would get done in a certain way, and if the expectations were not being met, we would have to part ways.

Going back to what I talked about earlier, asking questions is important. We'd ask questions, such as, "What's getting in your way of doing this? Why are you not able to get him out of bed? What is happening that you're not getting him to the day care facility on time? Or why are we feeding him cereal every morning when it's only on Saturday that he's scheduled to have cereal?" Yes, they were specific questions. They had to be to protect my dad's best interests.

Following up on the documentation we had in place helped us better understand what was going on with their days, too. We asked what their morning was like so we knew if they were running into specific problems for some reason or another. Texting back and forth with caregivers played a big role for caregiving for my dad. They would let us know if he didn't seem to be feeling well or let us know that they weren't sure it would be a good day for him to go out anywhere. Those kinds of conversations happened regularly. If there was a caregiver that couldn't or wouldn't do what we were asking, we were quick to ask for someone else. Yes, we had to train more people. This made things a bit more difficult, but we couldn't allow someone to continue to be with him whom we didn't trust or we didn't feel was doing the right thing on his behalf.

There were times when I heard the way a caregiver spoke to him or the way Dad responded to a caregiver that made me uncomfortable. We would let the company know that we no longer wanted that person, and we needed to find a replacement for them.

Each time we hired a company, there might be four to five employees that were on the team when they started out. They would be the ones who were trained and would be sharing shifts caring for my dad. As time went on and life happened, there would be a person that dropped off here or there.

We found that some companies were not willing to add someone new to take the place of the person who left. They would offer someone we were already using to have more hours, which was fine, except when that person was sick or something else happened that caused them to not come in for their shift. The main reason why most of those companies were fired was that our team would dwindle to such a point that we weren't confident or comfortable in the knowledge we'd have enough help when we needed it.

Trust Your Gut

If something doesn't feel right, it's probably not right. My dad and I were in business together at the time of his diagnosis. We owned a small company, and I learned a lot from him because he had extensive experience in many aspects of business. As an employer, I questioned my gut for many years. I've learned with Dad's encouragement, age, and wisdom that there's typically a reason why my gut is telling me something. Even if I can't put my finger on it, or even if I can logically talk myself out of it, I have learned that my gut is usually right.

You have to go with your gut
when you're hiring and firing people.

We would let the company know specifically what we were concerned about, whether it was an employee who needed to be replaced or the lack of a team big enough to handle what we needed. If they weren't willing to make the changes necessary, we just made the phone call and made a switch. Switching was harder for my sister than it was for me, because she was the one who was dealing with the phone calls. If someone wasn't going to show up to work, they weren't calling me since I was a state away; they were calling her because she lived only a few miles away from Dad. When we brought in a different company, she knew it would mean training a new company in how we wanted things done.

But that fear is not something that can get in the way. You really have to just make that step forward and know that it's going to be a better situation in the long run. The blessing was usually right around the corner; we just had to be willing to make that step to get there. We would work together as a team and get to that place where we could all be happy. Managing others is difficult.

When you think of all the hats that you're wearing as a caregiver when caring for a parent, often times you don't realize the boss hat is going to be one of those hats you're going to have to wear. I am hoping that as you read about some of what we went through, these tips and ideas will help you be more prepared for that role as you move into being the manager for the people who are caring for your parents.

There's a lot to think about in the functionality of taking care of an aging parent. This can be overwhelming if you're not prepared. I hope my story will go a long way in making sure you're as prepared as possible for everything that could happen around those corners. I want you to know, I do understand and you're not alone in this.

Notes

_____

_____

_____

_____

_____

_____

_____

_____

_____

_____

_____

_____

_____

_____

_____

_____

_____

_____

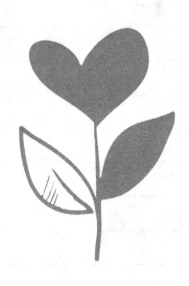

PART 2

Caring for Yourself

Dear Strong Daughter/Son,

You are doing great work. You are managing a lot right now. Take the time to assess how you are really doing.

You hear it all the time—because it's true—you must take care of you as well as take care of your parent. How are you doing at taking care of you?

Being strong doesn't mean neglecting your needs; it means taking the necessary steps to take care of yourself. You can have a full life while caring for your parent.

Rayna

CHAPTER 11

Understanding Your Needs

Sometimes, we forget there is more than one person that we're caring for in all of this. When in the middle of caring, we can allow the pressures of what we're doing, who we're doing it for, and the emotions we're experiencing overrun us, and that's something we have to be cautious of. The needs of those we're caring for usually get larger and larger and that makes us shrink the importance of taking care of ourselves. We actually stop paying attention to our own needs.

During the four-and-a-half-year period of caring for my dad, an area that really suffered for me was my eating habits. I took advantage of drive-throughs. In my everyday life, I live on a farm, so that's not an easy or a normal thing for me to do. But my dad lived in the city, so it got easier and easier to use the fast food drive-through. On top of eating more fast food, I didn't get the exercise I had been getting in the past. I didn't pay attention to myself like I should have. Needless to say, I put on extra weight.

*I found myself in a place where I realized
my weight was spinning out of control.*

I knew I needed to think about what I was doing for myself, and I had to be more intentional about it. I reached out to a friend and committed myself to a diet. I had previously tried different diet programs, which didn't work for me, but I thought, "Well, if it doesn't work, it doesn't work, but I'm going to give it an honest try."

The diet I chose was a wellness plan that included protein shakes. I wasn't sure I would be able to survive on protein meal replacements two times a day, but I gave it a try. Instead of driving through a fast food restaurant, I ate a protein bar and drank water during my drives. I replaced my breakfast with the nutrition in the shakes. To be honest, I did not want to give up all the things I enjoyed, so I splurged on my one "fork and knife meal" a day and continued to enjoy some of my favorite things. But as I saw the effort I was making pay off, I was motivated to try to eat healthier, even when I was eating out.

As I lost some of the weight, I felt I could make even better choices. I found a workout routine online that was fun, and I could do it in Dad's living room. I began to set goals for the number of steps I would get in each day, starting where I was and increasing a bit each week. Walking the stairs at Dad's was a great way to reach my goal, even if it was just before bed.

Over a nine-month period, I was able to lose sixty pounds. More importantly, I felt better and had more energy. In the midst of my caregiving season, putting the effort into taking care of myself made such a big difference for me.

Small steps resulted in a big change for me.

Like most things in life, we know the basics on what we need to do differently to get what we want, but we aren't willing to take those steps. In a caring season, your health is important, so I challenge you to do one thing today to help keep your body healthy and strong.

- Drink more water.
- Take one hundred more steps.
- Replace that high sugar snack with nuts or cheese.
- Get seven to eight hours of sleep.

You can do one thing, and I know that you will find you can do one more thing in just a few weeks.

As we find ourselves in this caregiving season, even those things that feel impossible can be tackled if we take it one step at a time. Focus on what needs to be done and understand your motivation for doing it. Taking care of yourself has to be on your list of things to do; in fact, it needs to be up at the top.

Self-awareness is key during this season.

There are some important things to understand as you're going through your season of caring. Because there will be a lot of stress on you, you need to:

- Take care of your body.
- Take care of yourself spiritually.
- Take care of your relationships.

There is a long list of subcategories that fall under those main points, but in essence, the lesson is that it's important to be paying close attention to yourself throughout this entire process.

Define Your Needs

Learning to define what your needs are will require you to think back to the things that bring you joy. I've talked about bringing joy to the one you are caring for, but you have to do the same thing for yourself. You might not have as much time to take part in those activities that you once did, but you still need to find out what they are.

One of my favorite things to do was play volleyball. With my travel schedule and all the other things on my plate, it really didn't work out for me to be able to continue to do that. While I couldn't play in that season, I needed to keep in mind it was something I could pick up later if I wanted to.

I love to sew, make crafts, crochet, and paint, so being creative was one thing I could do. As Dad went to bed early, 7:30 p.m. most nights, I could spend a couple of hours creating something. During the time I was with him, I took some online art courses, I took out my crochet hooks, and I even found a subscription program that sent a stamp project each month and got busy being creative. You can lose yourself in caregiving if you allow it, so taking care of yourself shouldn't be an option during this time. It's a must.

*Don't focus so much on their needs
that you forget about your own.*

Research tells us we are extremely sleep deprived in this country, and caregiving can multiply your chances of experiencing sleep deprivation exponentially. You need to think about how much sleep brings you refreshment. I'm an eight-hour-per-night kind of girl. If I don't get eight hours, I'm not very friendly or effective, especially in the morning. Sleep can be a real challenge with caregiving. It will make a big difference if you focus on getting the sleep your body requires.

*You have to do what you have to do
to make sure you stay at the top of your game.*

I had to find a way to carve out the time I needed and protect my sleep time to make sure that if I was in a season where my dad was not sleeping well, I still found a way to get the eight hours—taking naps when he was somewhere else or asking for help to cover a longer shift, so I could sleep in a little bit longer. Making adjustments to schedules—yours or others—is necessary at times.

Prioritize Relationships

Another area of priority has to be relationships—the relationships with your spouse, your kids, and your friends. Those people are the ones who support you and bring you joy in a totally different way. Make sure that you have these relationships set as priorities and you schedule time with these people.

I talked earlier about how I changed my schedule with my dad because my husband and I enjoyed our Sundays together. When I was first traveling and caring for my dad, I was staying with Dad through Sunday so I could attend church with him. Then a caregiver would come in and relieve me, and I would head home to the farm.

That didn't allow me to spend Sunday with my husband. After six months, when we did an evaluation meeting of how things were going, Sundays with my husband was something I missed. We made an adjustment, and I started traveling to Dad's earlier on Thursday and came home earlier on Sunday so that my husband and I were able to meet for church and then have the entire afternoon together. That was an important adjustment for the relationship with my husband. He now knew I was prioritizing him in my schedule.

You want your relationships to be healthy when this season of caring is over.

You can get so wrapped up, even lost, in what you're doing and who you're doing it for that sometimes, the other people you love, who are also needing your attention, get put on the backburner. In truth, you need attention from those relationships, as well. All relationships need nurture and care, so you run a real risk of putting yourself in a bad position if you dive too deeply into what you're doing for your parent and neglect some of those other important relationships that make you who you are.

Your overall wellbeing plays such an important role in your ability to give the type of care and attention you will need to give in any season of caring. Keeping a keen eye on how you are holding up is your responsibility. Caregiving can be very strenuous, both physically and mentally. There were times when I had to pick Dad up from the floor if he had fallen, or I got little sleep because he didn't want to go to bed, and that could be very exhausting.

Just as you have to build a detailed schedule of care for the person you are caring for, you have to expend that same effort in your own care. You may not immediately think about things like the conditions you are sleeping in when you are away from your home, or even little things like, how riding in the car a lot can cause issues with your hips or back.

Caregivers can have a difficult time understanding that their wellbeing is as important as the wellbeing of those they are caring for. Are you getting your doctor's appointments in and getting your eyes checked, your teeth cleaned? Those regular appointments are often the things people who are in a caregiving season allow to slide, and they can compound, causing a lot of problems later.

Knowing how you're doing emotionally is also important. We'll talk more about this later in the book, but there's a lot of grief that happens through the caregiving season, as you're watching your parents age. Your emotions will get out of whack. Examining why and taking some time to process through those emotions is an important thing to do for you.

For now, this is the new normal. Sometimes we wander into a caregiving season because we just find our parents need more and more. We want to maintain life as it always has been while adding on these additional responsibilities. Most of us are already busy. We are professionals with a job to take care of, as well as parents ourselves, with children and/or grandchildren to care for.

Dumping these additional responsibilities on top of an already full life really won't work.

It's important to think about the fact that there might be some things you'll need to let go of so that you can add these new responsibilities into your life. One of the ways you can do that is to be intentional about evaluating how you're doing.

Do Check-Ins with Yourself

In a structured way, have a regularly scheduled time to ask yourself some questions. I did mine on my drive back to the farm because I had almost four hours to think. I asked myself questions, which usually started with, "How was the weekend?" I had a rating system from one to ten—one being awful and ten being great. I rated how that weekend went, and then stopped to think specifically about what went well. Maybe it was bedtime, maybe it was the meals that I cooked, or maybe it was an activity that my dad and I were able to do.

I also thought about what did not go well, evaluating if we had a difficult time getting to bed or if he didn't sleep well or I didn't sleep well. I would contemplate about what it was that didn't go well and then ask myself, "What do I need to do differently for it to go better next time?"

Sometimes there wasn't anything I could do differently. It was just a situation that happened, but sometimes, there were things I knew I could do to help it go better next time.

I also asked that simple question, "How am I feeling?" Naming our emotions can help us get a better handle on what they are. Sometimes, I felt exhausted. Maybe I didn't get those eight hours of sleep during one or more of the nights. If that was the case, I planned to get a nap in during the week or go to bed earlier a few nights that week.

I love author Michele Cushatt's quote in her book, *Undone: A Story of Making Peace With an Unexpected Life.* "This is a rough-draft life. And whatever I didn't like about today, I can always edit tomorrow." There were times I just felt emotional. There might be something specific that happened, which caused me to be upset, or I might have felt frustrated with the help. Putting a label on that feeling helps us understand better what it is and clarify what edits we need to make for tomorrow. Being conscious of those things and intentionally addressing them can make a big difference.

Make sure that you're making a concentrated effort to focus in on the things that could be slipping by very easily.

It is such a busy season. There are always to-do lists with seemingly a million things, so if you aren't intentional with taking care of yourself, it will not make it to the list. You can make your list and know there are all these things that you need to do, but you do have to get to a point that you realize that there just might be some things you can't do. Be intentional with your needs and make sure you're taking care of those needs.

Know Your Limitations

There are limitations for every human being because there are only so many hours in the day. You can only have so much energy in this season of your life. You have to evaluate everything and know that while you can't do it all, you can do the things that are most important to you. Be honest with yourself, understand your feelings, and take the time to be able to do something besides take care of someone else.

When I left Dad's and came back to the farm, there were people at my home to take care of, too. It was easy to stay in caregiver mode. I had to know that I needed to plan fun. I needed to plan downtime. I needed to plan something other than taking care of someone else, and it was okay to do that.

Women generally feel guilty when they try to take care of themselves, but quite honestly, there's only so much of you. In order for you to be able to make it to the end of this journey, you are going to have to be a person who can say no to those things that cannot be a priority for you right now, during this season.

You have to be a person who is willing to look for help.

Widening your circle of support, finding a support group, so to speak, can really make a difference for you. Look at your faith community as an option, whether it's at your home or at the home of the person you're caring for.

People are always more willing to help when they realize there's a need, but often we don't bother to ask. If you think of a need and are willing to ask, you'd be surprised at the number of people willing to step forward and help, whether it's to pick up groceries or help pick up kids from school. Pay close attention to the fact that you do have needs, and you do have limitations. None of us like to admit this, but admitting it is the first step to getting the help you need.

Understanding your limitations helps you prioritize.

Sometimes, we get caught up in thinking something is too minor to ask someone else to help with, and we just figure on we'll do it ourselves. What we don't realize is how much time, effort, and energy it can take. Even just picking up something from the grocery store can be a challenge. The smallest bits of help can make a big difference to you. It's also okay to say, "No, I can't do this, someone else will need to take this on."

Know your limits, set your boundaries, and let others help with the things you can't or don't want to do.

When I started staying with my dad, he was the only person living in his home. One of the things I laid out as a boundary for myself was that I didn't want to do the grocery shopping. I already grocery shopped for my family when I was there during half the week. I didn't want to spend my "dad time" grocery shopping, too. I had to set that boundary. I knew it would cause me a lot of frustration, and it would have been very draining to me.

But we had to figure out who would do the grocery shopping. In this day and age, shopping can be done online, which is so much easier than navigating grocery store aisles. Now, I know grocery shopping sounds like such a minor thing with everything else you're going to be dealing with, but think about the time it takes, the effort it takes to do the inventory and make the list, then the unloading and putting away the groceries when you get home. That's time that could be spent on other, important things.

Your Rest and Relaxation

I just talked about how getting my rest in this season was important to me. In general, life can be draining, but when you're caring for the needs of someone else, it can be that much more exhausting. It's crucial to focus not just on what time you go to bed, but your quality of sleep. There are some great apps available that can help you monitor how well you're sleeping. I have an Android phone, so I used the "Sleep for Android" app in conjunction with my Galaxy watch. It was fascinating to see how much deep sleep I got one night as compared to another.

From the start, Dad was up and down a lot to use the restroom during the night. I've always been a sound sleeper. It concerned me that he was getting up in the middle of the night because there were times that I did not hear him. That concern caused me to be hyper-vigilant, waking up with every little noise. I struggled with not feeling rested.

We needed to adjust something so I could get the rest I needed. We purchased a bed alarm. Any time my dad's weight was off the bed, the alarm would sound. I knew that would wake me up for sure. That gave me the confidence I needed to not worry about every little noise

I heard through the night. With the alarm, I knew when he was out of bed and could go in and check on him.

Simple things like evaluating what's affecting your sleep will be helpful. Realize that rest is not only about sleep, but it's the ability to feel rested within your soul and your body, which means being able to step away momentarily.

You can feel like it's unrealistic to get away and get out of the caring routine. Just like a vacation from a job, taking a break from caregiving can let you come back more rested and ready to jump right back in.

Taking respite breaks can make all the difference in the world in a caring season.

The first year that we were caring for Dad in his home, I was there fifty out of fifty-two weekends, and that was a lot. At one of our official sit-downs to evaluate how things were going, I expressed concern that I was missing out on time with my family. I wanted to figure out if there was a way I could get a weekend off a month. In the second year, we figured out a way to get me that weekend a month.

Whether it was my grandson's birthday party or an event with my husband, with an adjustment, I was able to start participating in family events again. We were able to bring somebody else in to cover the time I was away. It really did rejuvenate me and helped me make it the full four and a half years.

Rest looks different for different people. Someone who is an introvert gets energy by being alone. Once your energy's been sapped, you have to recharge by being by yourself. If you're an extrovert, you need to be around other people, so you recharge by interacting with others. If you're an extroverted person and you're stuck at home caregiving for someone, you're probably feeling pretty drained if you aren't getting out and around other people. You have to consider what makes you feel rested and what you need to feel refreshed and ready to go.

As an introvert going through a stressful situation, I needed quiet time, completely alone, to recharge. Without it, it was easy to start shutting down and not be effective in providing the care necessary for this season. Being aware of this helped me realize I needed to take advantage of the time when Dad went to bed early. Instead of filling my time with television or even visiting on the phone with a friend I need to rest and recharge. Getting the time by myself to think and relax helped me do a better job.

When caregiving, you feel like you can't afford to do things for yourself, but the reality is that you can't afford not to.

To honor our parents and love them well, we have to be at our best, and we have to figure out a way to be able to show up as the best version of ourselves as possible. Know your needs, know your limitations, and get the rest you need. Take the time to make *you* a priority, and you will be able to show up in a better, more equipped way to give the care needed in this season.

Notes

Dear Loyal Daughter/Son,

I know it is hard to imagine life without your parent, but there will be a day when they are no longer here. You will do all that you can to walk them all the way home, and you will live on as their legacy.

This season feels like it will never end, but I promise, it will seem too short when the day arrives when they are no longer here.

Your parent wants you to take care of you while caring for him/her. They want you to nurture your marriage and other important relationships while you nurture them. They love you and always, always will.

Rayna

CHAPTER 12

Don't Forget About Life After This Season

There are times you will feel this season is never going to end. The truth is, it will come to an end. This time is about walking your parent home and doing so with no regrets.

I challenge you to intentionally think about a time when this season will be over. Unless you're thinking big picture and planning accordingly, then you might find yourself completely lost once this season is over. Whether you want to think about it or not, you need to.

If you don't, not only will you have to deal with the grief of losing your parent, but you'll have lost just about everything else, as well. Most of the time, if people don't plan for the end, then they probably haven't maintained their life well while caring for their parent. In order for that not to happen, you have to see the big picture and think through what is important for you at the end of this.

*What are the most important things in your life
that you want to still have once the season is over?*

Caregiving is a demanding job, but you don't have to give up everything just to be a person who honors, loves, and cares for an aging parent. Take some time to consider the impact caregiving can have on each of these areas of your life. Then make a plan to ensure you have the relationships in your life that are most important.

Don't Give Up Friendships

Without realizing it, you might find yourself too busy to get together with friends. You may be cutting conversations shorter than usual or not reaching out at all. Friendships, like all relationships, require a time commitment. Your time together might need to look different than it used to, but remember, your friendships provide an important benefit to your life.

One of the things I did was have regular lunch or dinner dates with friends. It might not have been as often as what it was before I was traveling to spend time with my dad, but it was definitely important to have them on my calendar. Planning ahead and blocking that time to meet a friend for lunch, go to a painting class, take a walk, or do a Bible study were all things I enjoyed with friends during my season of caring. Doing the things, you enjoy with the people you love helps maintain those relationships so that they're still strong when this season is over.

Even if you don't think you have the time, you can pick up the phone and have a conversation. I may not have gotten the face-to-face time with my friends as often as before, but I still took the time to stay in touch with them.

Your Spiritual Health

Not only did I keep myself emotionally and physically strong, but I had to keep myself spiritually strong to deal with everything that was happening in my season. One of the things I found that worked really well for me was an online Bible study.

I had taught Bible study and was involved with groups of women studying the Bible together, but in this season the face-to-face time didn't work. I needed to make an adjustment to still feed myself spiritually. Being able to have a spiritual life that's strong and to continue past the season of caring meant that I had to find a way to do it during this season, as well.

I found Proverbs 31 and Lifeway online Bible studies to be two of my favorite resources. I also lead book studies through my company, Take Heart Coaching. Connecting with women all over the states to learn and grow in our faith is a blessing that fed my soul for sure.

Career Adjustment

I mentioned early on in this book that I had made an adjustment in my career during my season of caring. I had closed our business and moved to the farm on a full time basis eighteen months before the need for me to become a hands-on caregiver for Dad arrived. At that point, I was teaching four half-days a week at a local elementary school.

I loved being able to give the kids the skills they needed to be more successful in school, but I also loved working with the parents. Offering a listening ear, resource, and advice was a very rewarding part of my job at the learning center we owned. I missed being able to impact the families when I went back to teaching in a traditional setting.

After exploring career options, I discovered Life Coaching and began classes to receive my Certified Professional Life Coach credential. I was able to arrange my classes so I could continue my studies while teaching and caring for Dad. After the first six months, I knew I wanted to continue to care for Dad in his home, and my sister and husband were on board, too. But juggling it all was too much; I knew that. I was ready to let go of the teaching position and launch Take Heart Coaching. My coaching is done over the phone or video chat, so it was a perfect fit for me in this season.

Is there a way for you to work online or change how you work in order to continue your current career and take care of your parents? Sometimes you can maintain your job through your season of caring, but sometimes you can't. It's not always an easy adjustment, but there are ways to integrate caring into your career.

Grieve Often

During this season, you have to be willing to grieve. Emotions can feel big and overwhelming. It can feel like it's too much to allow yourself to sit with your grief. If you don't deal with that grief throughout the season, you're going to find yourself overcome with it at the end of the season.

Sitting in the grief—allowing yourself to identify what it is that's bringing that grief on in the moment or shortly after, can remind you that you have a life you still love and can come back to after your season of caring for your parent.

Sometimes, we feel like allowing ourselves to grieve in the moment is a sign of weakness. We feel we don't have time for that or can't allow that to take place. The reality is, there's a level of strength we draw from allowing ourselves to deal with those emotions, by allowing that grieving process to happen, even in the midst of the season.

Grieving in the moment is going to be different then grieving once they're gone.

The things you'll grieve when they're gone might be things like not having a hug or hearing their voice again. The grieving in these caregiving moments will be for things, such as them not being able to be your parent in the same way they had in the past or for their loss of independence.

This is a season and it will come to an end, and the next season will have to be lived out.

Not grieving in the season can make it harder to deal with your family and loved ones, too. There will be many levels of bereavement. To avoid grief in the moment definitely brings heavier, harder, and longer periods of grief after they're gone. I promise, this is something that will help when this season is over. It's a powerful way to set yourself up so that when this season comes to an end and the new season starts, you can move forward well.

It's a Marathon

Caring for your aging parent is not a short-term process. It isn't a sprint. It's not something that you're going to rush through to get it done. This is a process that could take some time. When raising children, they get older and they become more independent. For the most part, you know when they're going to be leaving the house. There's a typical timeline you can track.

When you're journeying with your parents to the end, the process is the opposite. They are becoming more and more dependent on you. It's difficult to know just how long that journey will be. My sister and I looked at each other more than once and said, "I can't believe we're still doing this." When I first approached her, I asked her if we could do this for six months. Our season ended at four and a half years.

There is no way to have control over when the season will come to an end. You will want to control it, but you must make it a priority to care for yourself so that you know you'll be a strong source of support all the way through to the end, even when you don't know how long the marathon will be.

Make New Decisions

Realize that with each step of the way, you're just doing the best you can do. Sometimes it feels like you're making these big decisions that you can't unmake. Adopting the mentality that every decision is not permanent, but rather, you can decide to make a new decision at any time will help you make decisions throughout the journey all the way to the end.

I talked about how for the first year I was with my dad fifty out of fifty-two weekends. After our family talk before that second year, I was at Dad's about forty weekends. By the third year, I was closer to thirty-six, and by the fourth year, I needed to drop to every other weekend.

As time went along, it was still really important for me to be there and be with him, but I also found it became harder, both emotionally and physically, to care for his needs. I needed more time off, which meant we added more support into the process. Aunt Colleen, who had lived with my dad before he progressed to where he needed constant care, was able to do a few nights a week for the first couple of years, but then she found herself in a place where it became too much for her also. It's what works best for "right now" and when it stops working, you can make a new decision.

There are times that we think a decision we make is going to impact the situation in such a way that it's going to be unfixable. We fear it's going to change things to a point that we can't come back from it. It's freeing to make the decision and understand that if you don't like the results, you can make another choice.

No decision has to be a forever decision.

Make the best decision you can for right now and give yourself permission to make a new one if you need to. That's a really powerful way of reframing a lot of the overwhelm that comes with trying to make the best decisions for our loved one.

Notes

_____

_____

_____

_____

_____

_____

_____

_____

_____

_____

_____

_____

_____

_____

_____

_____

Dear Amazing Daughter/ Son,

There will be days when you feel there is no way you can keep doing all that you are doing. That is completely normal, but that does not make it true. You will need rest here and there, and that is okay. You will also need to learn to say no.

Learning who you are and what is most important to you will make knowing when to say yes and when to say no easier.

Invest in discovering your values so you can live by them with ease.

Rayna

CHAPTER 13

Keep Things Running Smoothly

I talked about the importance of keeping the life of the one you are caring for running smoothly, but keeping things running smoothly for yourself is no less important. It's definitely going to be a challenge, but it's extremely important that your life stay as normal as possible.

I have used the word intentional quite a bit in this book. That word keeps coming up because it is the one word you must keep in mind during this caring season. Your life was full before you started this season, and it's about to get even fuller.

Without a clear intention to keep your life moving smoothly for you, it could get real difficult real fast.

I was able to maintain a lot of how my life was before this season of caring started, and I was even able to add to my life during it.

- I changed my entire professional career by finishing my life coach training.
- I established Take Heart Coaching, my business.
- I became a grandma.
- I started a web design business as well.

There were a lot of pieces added to my life throughout my caring season. To do that smoothly, I had to plan ahead and use my time wisely.

Your life should never be on autopilot during your season of caring. There are ways of making sure your life can run smoothly and avoid tripping yourself up as you go through this process, and autopilot is not one of them; it's not realistic.

This is a time you need to be very self-aware. None of us make good decisions in the thick of emotion or overwhelm. Otherwise, we make reactionary decisions. A reaction is really not a decision. People who make decisions based on reaction tend to overreact. When we make a decision without overreacting, we are actually taking control of our ability to think through the decision.

When feeling emotional, our brain shuts down our ability to think. It goes into reaction mode, choosing between fight, flight, or freeze. When emotions are overtaking us, we don't have the ability to think clearly, and that's why reactive decisions don't make sense.

Decisions should only be made from a calm place.

Take the time to talk through the decisions that need to be made. Write out your pros and cons for that decision. Educate yourself with all the information you need to make a solid decision. Don't forget to view the decision in light of your core values. It can make a huge difference in what you decide. During this season, simple decisions can feel huge. Rather than wandering aimlessly, have confidence that you're living in a way that's aligned with your values by taking the time to make decisions from a serene place. I have added a resource for this in the back of the book.

A Personal Manifesto

I was excited to find a book called *Overwhelmed* written by Kathi Lipp and Cheri Gregory early in my caring season. The authors talked about the process of writing a personal manifesto, and it made all the difference in my life. It helped me live by my priorities so that I could have a life to walk back into after this season ended.

In general, a personal manifesto is a written statement, which includes your core values. The great thing about these statements is they might not be completely true about you today, but your desire is for them to be true of you at the end of this season.

A personal manifesto functions as your own personal code of conduct that is not decided in the moment but predetermined before you are in crisis.
—Kathi Lipp

These are statements about who you are and what's important to you in your life before you find yourself in the midst of decisions that will either support or contradict the things you say are most important to you.

By writing your manifesto, you have guidelines that will assist you in making the best decisions possible. The process of the manifesto is really quite simple. You think about what you treasure most. What are your core values? What do you think is most important? Identify five to eight of those core values, and turn them into statements that will provide guidance on how you will live them out. If you need help determining your core values, visit the resources in the back of the book to learn more about how to do this.

Writing a manifesto will help you to think through those things that are most important and help you mold your life in such a way that you're living according to those principles. I found it really helpful to put myself in the future and think about what I wanted people to say about me when I'm no longer here. I want to be true to who God made me to be, and I want to be true to the mission that He put on my heart. Here is my first manifesto.

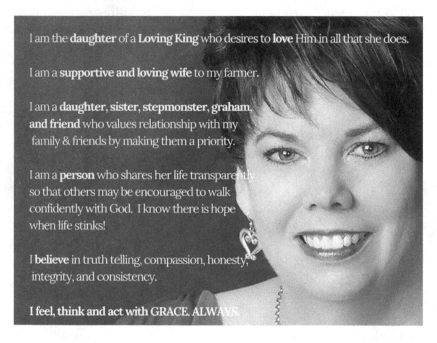

I am the **daughter** of a **Loving King** who desires to **love** Him in all that she does.

I am a **supportive and loving wife** to my farmer.

I am a **daughter, sister, stepmonster, graham, and friend** who values relationship with my family & friends by making them a priority.

I am a **person** who shares her life transparently so that others may be encouraged to walk confidently with God. I know there is hope when life stinks!

I **believe** in truth telling, compassion, honesty, integrity, and consistency.

I feel, think and act with GRACE. ALWAYS.

I started off with a statement. *I am a daughter of the loving King.* One of the things I emphasized was that loving part because in this season of my life, things were hard. It was difficult to watch my dad changing and at times, I questioned God's love. It was important for me to make the statement (a reminder to myself) that He is loving, and I know that I love Him. I want to live that way.

I am a supportive and loving wife to my farmer. I knew that even though I wasn't home with him all the time, I wanted to remind myself to always be supportive of him and what he did on the farm, as well as loving him well, showing and expressing that love every time I had the chance.

The third statement was *I'm a daughter, sister, stepmonster, graham, and friend who values relationship with my family and friends by making them a priority.* I wanted to list out those different roles. We jokingly call me the stepmonster. The kids don't really think that, but it adds humor in there, and graham is my grandma name.

I wanted to list the people who were important to me, so as I read that statement, family and friend's faces come to mind. I think about how important they are to me. And so, I make it a point to make those people a priority by spending time with them and investing in their lives.

The next statement, *I am a person who shares her life transparently so that others may be encouraged to walk confidently with God. I know there is hope when life stinks.* The mission of my coaching practice when I first started was to help people walk through transitions and find God faithful through that time. That sentence was one that expressed my heart to help people see that even when life is hard, there's hope in Him.

And then *I believe in truth telling, compassion, honesty, integrity, and consistency.* These were some of the characteristics about me that I wanted to continue to live out. I wanted to be a person who could speak truth to those caregivers in my life when needed. I wanted to be compassionate and honest with others, and consistency and integrity have always been important core values for my life.

And as for the last piece of my manifesto, that year, God gave me the word grace, so *I think, feel, and act with grace—always.* That was a statement that probably wasn't always true about me, but definitely one He reminded me of throughout that year. I grew in grace toward others when they weren't doing exactly what I thought they should do. This allowed me to remember that I needed to focus on the grace. I also needed to learn to extend myself more grace. As a person who has high standards for herself, learning to extend grace to myself in every circumstance helped.

This process was very impactful for me through this season of caring, and I took these words and put them on a photo of myself, which I love, and I hung it in my office. Often times, I read through it to remind myself of who I am and how I was created so that I am able to be faithful to my mission and pre-decide those things that might get a little blurry during struggles and challenges.

I loved having my personal manifesto on that picture of myself because I could revisit those statements in that light and know that's the person behind this mission. Most of us don't like the way we look in pictures. We look at our flaws, but when I saw that particular picture, I said, "That's me. That's who I am." That's the image I wanted to see when I read those statements. This is who God made me to be, and I can stand true to that. It allowed me to remember who I was in moments I might have otherwise forgotten in that overwhelming season.

Put your personal manifesto somewhere where you can see it constantly so that you never lose sight of who you are going into a caring season, and you'll still know who you are coming out.

Some of the statements, I was able to live out pretty well at that point, but others were definitely areas where I knew I needed to grow. It reminded me to live intentionally and keep my priorities clear, even in the face of everything else that happens in life. Over the years, I have taken the time to update and edit my manifesto as things have changed in my life.

Pre-Decide

Pre-deciding is another concept taught in the book *Overwhelmed*. Learning to make decisions before you find yourself in the heat of the moment is pre-deciding. One of the things I appreciate about my manifesto is that it pre-decides for me. There are so many good opportunities that we're provided, but if we say yes to everything, we find ourselves stretched way too thin, preventing us from giving our best to anyone.

I was able to use this in situations, such as when someone asked if I could help teach Sunday School at church. When I considered that request against my personal manifesto, it was an easy decision. It definitely lined up with serving God, which is one of the first things listed, but would it have allowed me to be a supportive and loving wife? Would it have allowed me to be a sister and a daughter and a grandparent?

At that season in life, there wasn't enough of me to do all of those things and love on a room full of little kiddos at Sunday School, too. I had to pass on that opportunity at that moment but knew I could come back to it in another season. Allowing my manifesto to govern my calendar has helped me for many years.

Each January, I revisit and rewrite some items, add new things, or edit others. It gives me a chance to look at the areas of growth (good) or the areas of new focus that God is bringing into my life, ensuring that they're on my priority list.

Manifestos open up different opportunities for you to know how to move forward because you have it on paper. Your personal manifesto is your benchmark, one you can leverage to make some of those tough decisions and make them quickly. It really allows you to live with no regrets, because you do spend the time processing and thinking through what is most important and understanding that your time and resources are limited in this season. (You can learn more about writing your own personal manifesto on the resource page at the end of this book.)

Lysa TerKeurst addresses the concept of learning when to say yes and when to say no in her book *The Best Yes: Making Wise Decisions in the Midst of Endless Demands*. She reminds us that saying yes to something means there is less of you—less time, less energy, and just less for other things. Realize your yes has consequences, and be sure what you say yes to be worth the tradeoff—less of you in return.

If you have pre-decided, then you don't have to feel guilty about saying no to opportunities that come along.

You can increase your ability to focus and be confident in who you are and what's most important to you. As you navigate this season, make sure that you keep yourself as part of the forefront of your care. This will help you realize that it's okay to live in a way that you don't regret allowing the good things to distract you from the best things in order to keep your life running smoothly.

Notes

_____

_____

_____

_____

_____

_____

_____

_____

_____

_____

_____

_____

_____

_____

_____

_____

Dear Emotional Daughter/Son,

It is normal to feel emotional during this season that is filled with many small losses. You are able to feel the grief and the joy at the same time—you really can.

Your loneliness is normal. No one knows exactly what you are feeling during this season. Don't let that stop you from sharing with others who are in a common season.

Remember to focus on all the things you have to be thankful for. Even in this season, they are always there.

Rayna

CHAPTER 14

Dealing with Obstacles

Emotions are running high throughout this season of caring. Our feelings get intense, and sometimes, total emotional exhaustion can set in. I would say the biggest emotion I experienced through my season of caring was grief.

Grief is a daily part of caregiving—at least it should be. Watching a loved one decline is not easy, and witnessing them not being able to do things that used to be easy and natural for them is sad. It is also difficult to let go of the relationship we once had with our loved one. Grief is natural with loss, and it helps if we don't hold all of that grief in until the end of the journey. You have to deal with it in the moment.

Even though I'd been through this season with my mom and had grieved things she wasn't able to do, it was different with my dad. I was still an adolescent when Mom was diagnosed, and the changes in who she was and what she was able to do—as far as communicating and caring for herself—came very quickly in her illness.

Losing my mom was certainly a loss, but it was more about the loss of all the things I didn't have with her. With Dad, that loss was continual throughout his gradual decline. It was the loss of what was and what we were able to do in our relationship. It was the loss in communication we had. Dad had always been the person I ran to in my life. He was always such a big supporter, even throughout my adult life, so this loss was really intense.

It surprised me how intense my grief was after losing him physically. The intensity of the grief was shocking. This was not just sadness, which is what we often think of with grief. Beyond the sadness, the "fog" that comes with having a life-changing event was massive. My ability to concentrate and focus was missing.

After saying goodbye to my dad, the changes in my life were immense. My schedule opened up, and all of this time I had been spending with Dad was now available. I thought I would be able to take advantage of that time and move into developing my business and focus on other parts of my life.

In reality, I really needed time to grieve, time to be sad, and time to process it all. After he passed, we also had to deal with the family home. It had been in our family for forty-three years. Packing that up and getting it ready to sell was a deep loss. We had roots there, and that house had always been a safe place to return to when life was not what I expected.

Grief is definitely one of the biggest obstacles through the season, as well as after the season is over.

In *Understanding Your Grief: Ten Essential Touchstones for Finding Hope and Healing Your Heart*, Alan Wolfelt talks about grief in a way I found really helpful. Sometimes you can't understand death, especially a death of someone that you've loved so deeply. Not being able to understand it really causes you to struggle and wrestle with the mystery of death—why people die and what happens through death.

Stages of Grief

We've all heard of the stages of grief. We want grief to be clean and easy, and we want to take the mystery out of *it*. The sad thing is that's really not the way it works.

We have misapplied those stages of grief. Elisabeth Kubler-Ross introduced the concept of the stages of death in 1969. Denial, anger, bargaining, depression, and acceptance are the five stages we are all likely familiar with.

We expect our grief to walk right down that linear path, experiencing each of the feelings, finally reaching acceptance, and moving on with our lives. But Kubler-Ross never intended for those stages to be interpreted as rigid, linear stages that all people experience in the same way. Rather, she developed this concept of stages for terminally ill patients to help them understand the experiences *they* will have with grief because of *their* terminal illness.

As a culture, we have interpreted her work to mean that all of us will feel the same in our mourning. Because of this, people struggle through the grief season because they feel like they should just be experiencing each of those stages individually and then close the door on those feelings and move to the next one. In reality, a lot of the feelings are going to be simultaneous and last for different lengths of time. Each person's grief is unique; don't make the mistake of trying to pinpoint exactly where you should be in the stages, but rather allow yourself to naturally be where you are.

There will be a blurring of stages and emotions with grief.

I would recommend that while you're in the process of caring for your parent, remember that grief is a normal part of what you're experiencing. The roles that you've played in the past are not the same now, and they're not going to be the same in the future. That's going to cause you to experience grief. Go ahead and feel it, name it, and allow it to be a part of the process.

Also remember, just because you grieve while you're caring for your parent, it doesn't protect you from the grief that's going to come once they're gone. Those expectations can really impact how hard it hits you, so know going in this is going to be intense throughout and after this season ends.

Of course, it's not the same for everybody. The way my sister grieved, and the way that I grieved was very different and that's okay. You have to grieve for the amount of time you need to grieve, and you need to be open to allowing those around you to do the same.

Learning how to grieve for who your parent no longer is can cause a lot of emotions to come up. Grief and emotions are never set in stone. They impact each person differently and come in waves. Often, we try to mask them and push them down, but that causes even more issues. If you are able to experience that grief through the process, I promise it will help.

It's important to become aware of what the source of your emotional response is. When I was caring for my dad, and he wasn't able to do something he had always been able to do before, that caused my frustration to rise. My expectation was that he could do that task.

The frustration isn't really about what we're trying to accomplish right now, but rather with the result not being what we expected—things are not what they've always been before. My frustration was coming from me seeing and realizing that my dad just couldn't do the things he could do before. For me, any time there was great emotion in the moment, I needed to step back and realize where that emotion was coming from.

Most of the time, my emotional response was coming from grief over what was no longer.

In running our business together, there were conversations about the books or the bills or trying to make decisions on investments, with advertising, and eventually, all of those things became difficult.

When I asked Dad questions, his answers became more and more vague. He would start to repeat the information I was giving him. He reached a point where he could no longer participate in problem-solving activities required to run the business. He just couldn't have those conversations with me anymore. That was a point of grief for me—realizing the business relationship we had was no longer one we could continue to have.

I wished it was different, but that is where we were. I couldn't continue to put him in a place where he was uncomfortable, trying to give me answers he didn't have or understanding something he could no longer understand. Letting go of that allowed us both to have more peace and enjoy what we could, which was being in the moment and appreciating the experiences that came with that.

It's important to realize grief might be the root cause of our emotions, which might seem out of whack for any given situation.

Realize what you're feeling and then look a little deeper to see where the emotion is coming from. You'll want to do this throughout your season, each time you feel those feelings where you are missing who they were and the relationship you had. Not identifying grief but instead, stuffing it down or ignoring it will make emotions more intense, especially in the end.

Grief is harder than one might think; it's a lot of work. If you take it a little bit at a time, it's easier to handle than if you allow it to overwhelm you in the end. Being able to work through these emotions along the way will help get you to that point where you can deal with it as it comes, as opposed to have it build up to be released all at one time.

Loneliness
When a parent is gone, there can be a lot of loneliness, no matter how great the rest of your family is and how much they are there for you.

It can almost feel like a sense of abandonment, as though you're an orphan. In my coaching, this has come up from time to time, especially when the last parent is gone. It really impacts us. Usually, when people refer to that, I often hear them say they know they're the next in line. The death of a parent causes many people to consider their own mortality.

When I lost my dad, the best way I can describe it was a feeling of being untethered. He was my grounding spot. He was the one I could always, always come back to. He was there through every season and phase of my life. Your parents are the only ones that have always been there with you. They're your home base, and now they're not there anymore. Understand that aspect of grief is likely going to be part of what you experience when you lose a parent.

There is going to be an intense loneliness when your parent is no longer there.

No one can look at his or her children without bias. Of course, we see the faults in our kids but nothing like what the rest of the world sees. The love we have for our children is uniquely different and so intense that we really can't see them with an open mind. For me, it was that realization that there was no one left on earth that sees me that way. Parents are the only ones that love us that deeply. There is a normalcy in understanding that these intense feelings are part of the grief that happens when you lose both of your parents.

How you respond to that grief also changes whether you're able to re-establish yourself and understand that they were important and their love was different than anybody else's love for us. Just because they're gone doesn't mean that's gone. Your parents have always loved and cherished you, and just because they're no longer here, it doesn't change who they've always been and who you've been to them.

When someone you love dies, you don't just lose
the presence of that person. As a result of the death,
you may lose many other connections to yourself
and the world around you.
—Alan Wolfelt

Loss can change a lot of things. You might feel like part of you has died. Part of my identity was tied to being a daughter. There is no one else in this world who calls me daughter, so that was something I had to grieve.

If you aren't careful, grief can lower your self-esteem and confidence. It can affect your health and even your personality; you may just not feel like yourself because of this great loss. You can experience a loss of emotional security because the support that only they can give is no longer there. This can also bring a loss of dreams or goals. It can challenge your faith or even trigger depression that causes you to lose your joy. While all of those things can be effects of grief, they don't have to be. Grief is the process of helping you integrate that loss into your life.

There is a *before*, but there will be an *after*. When you learn to integrate that loss into your life and take it as it comes, you will continue to have a life you can love. You will be happy again. Living with grief is just a season, much like the season of caring.

Emotions

There are many emotions you will encounter during in this season. It's totally natural to feel overwhelmed. You will feel like there's more to do than there is time, and that's okay. A lot of negative emotions that you might not expect may show themselves during this season. This is normal and natural.

Negative emotions creep in from being in a situation with multiple stressors. Being able to name and deal with those negative emotions is the first step in realizing they are the root cause of some of your thoughts and behaviors.

None of us want to admit when we're feeling jealous. In the season of caring for your parent, you are sacrificing, and you are giving up things that you see others having. You might not have spent as much time with the others whom you love. Thoughts like, "Why do I have to do everything? Why can't someone else help me more?" will come up.

Every time you head to social media, you get to see the best of everybody else's life. Maybe they're free to go on vacation more. You'll see them spending more time doing things that you used to love to do, and you just can't do them now. Jealousy can rear its ugly head, so you really have to focus on the moment and the joy that you have with the person you're taking care of to keep you from immersing yourself in those negative feelings.

Find a way to be grateful for what you have right now, whatever that might be.

There's going to be a time when this season is over. There will be more opportunities to do those things, which you might be wishing you could do right now, but there won't be more time and opportunity to develop new memories with your parents.

One of my favorite things to think about was the opportunity to sing with my parents. Both of them loved Nat King Cole, and we spent many hours listening to him and singing along to the songs. I was able to get a lot of hugs during that time—hugs I no longer have now that they are gone. Replace that jealousy with thankfulness for the moments you get to create with your parent.

Caregiver's Guilt

As a caregiver, our heart is with the one we are taking care of—always—but it's not healthy for us to be with them all the time. Being away from them can bring guilt because we're having somebody else do something that we feel like we should be doing.

There can be guilt from feeling we aren't doing enough for our parent; guilt could also come from wanting the season to be over. Because it's not a finite amount of time, we don't know where the finish line is, it can feel totally overwhelming and like the season is going to go on forever. The thought of, "When mom or dad isn't here anymore, I'll be able to do that again," can bring a ton of guilt.

Feeling like you don't love your loved one enough can bring on guilt; your impatience with them can usher in those guilty feelings. Not being with your husband or your grandkids or at that ballgame with your child brings feelings of guilt for caregivers. Realize that it's somewhat normal to feel guilty for those things.

Learning to silence the "shoulds" will make a big difference.

I should be here, I should do that, or *I should be able to handle this better.* When you start telling yourself these "shoulds," it's like saying you're not enough. That is a lie. What you're doing is important! You're doing a great job and you're doing the best you can and that's all you or anyone else can ask of you.

If you can identify when it's guilt that's making you feel bad, you can stop it and tell yourself, "All right, I am doing the best I can do." Look at it from a different perspective. This is how you can start dealing with those guilty feelings and moving out of condemnation and the realization that you're making a big difference to your parents. Don't allow yourself to dwell in the guilt.

Ignoring emotions will affect us emotionally and physically. The physical effects manifest through body aches, insomnia, loss of appetite, weight gain, or just an overall feeling of dreariness. Those emotions need to be dealt with, and if they aren't dealt with, it can lead to depression, which has even more physical ramifications. Emotions are one of the biggest obstacles you will deal with in your caregiving season. It's important we face all of the emotions we don't like to feel or talk about or even admit we have.

New life can grow, and I can see evidence of that fact. But
new life can grow only as it is watered by grief's tears.
—Michele Cushatt, *Relentless*

Negative emotions can definitely get in the way during this season, whether it's jealousy, grief, loneliness, or any other unwanted emotion. Name that emotion and don't let it overcome you. Pushing through those emotions is how you're going to get through this season and maintain your sanity and wellbeing.

Notes

Dear Resilient Daughter/Son,

You are stronger when you don't try to stand alone. Learn to say yes to help from others and to taking care of you.

It will be uncomfortable at first to accept help, but you will be surprised what a blessing it can be to both you and the person you are helping.

You are stronger when you learn to take care of you during this season. It won't come naturally; you will need to work at it, but I know you can do it.

Most of all, you have to hold on to hope in order to stay strong. Look for the hope, even in seasons of pain.

Rayna

CHAPTER 15

You Are Not Alone

Feeling lonely? I've touched on loneliness several times because it's important to know that everyone will experience this differently in his or her season. My story won't be your story, but the crucial thing you must know is that you are not alone.

While I had a great family support system, I know it won't look like that for everyone. Through my coaching, I have seen countless ways people have found the support they needed. When you are going through this yourself, just know there are many others dealing with a similar situation. A report released by The National Alliance for Caregiving (NAC) and AARP called "Caregiving in the U.S. 2020," and published in NAC's website showed there were almost fifty-three million family caregivers. These are people who were not paid caregivers but family members caring for a loved one just like you. Those numbers are a clear indication that you are not alone.

Support Groups

Many are walking this season alone and looking for others to come alongside. It's important to look for a support group and find encouragement from people who understand where you are. In this day and age, the Internet has amazing opportunities for online support groups. There are places to find information and connect with organizations that offer support. There are toll-free numbers to call and talk to someone if you're feeling at your wit's end. Finding what's available to you is easier than you realize.

Isolation can hit hard with caregiving, but there is support out there.

If possible, I recommend getting involved in an in-person, local support group. Taking the step to look for a support group can often feel overwhelming. You may be inclined to think, "I don't know any of these people. What will they think of me?" It may feel uncomfortable in the beginning, but there's something special about connecting with others who are on similar journeys.

I lead a support group once a month for family caregivers, and it's always such a joy when someone new joins us because we know we can welcome them and love on them and give them what they need. Know that when you're looking for your support group and make that step to walk in that room, people are going to be really excited to see you. The thing is, you may even be an answer to prayer for someone who's already involved in that group.

When an in-person group is not possible, there are online opportunities. Some sites have chat options where you can type back and forth with people. Some online support groups meet on a conference call or a videoconference system. I have a free support group that meets through videoconference each month. You can gather with other daughters who are in their seasons of caring to transparently share joys and struggles. You'll find understanding, support, and encouragement as you journey through this time if you allow others to be a part of your support team. There are even coaching groups available. When you join a coaching group, you develop relationships with others who are in a season of caring, too. You can find resources, friendships, and an even deeper level of support.

> **Locating Local Support Groups**
> Call 211 or go to 211.org
> Your local United Way
> Your local Agency on the Aging
> Alz.org
> Cancer.org
> ALSA.org
> DefeatDiabetes.org
> NourishforCaregiver.com
> Search Facebook for many options

Finding others outside your family who can support you can build a whole different layer of support that can make a huge difference.

What's great about bringing people together in a group setting, whether in person or online, is that we're in a common season, but we're not in the same places within that season. Being able to share your experiences and encourage others brings great joy. Having a variety of people who are in the same season helps you experience purpose, and you're able to say, "I've been there. I've learned that, and now I can share it with you."

Learn to Say Yes

There are people who are just natural caregivers. They will often say yes to diving in and helping other people without question, but one of the things that these caregivers will often have a hard time with is saying yes when someone offers to help them. Realizing you can only do so much is the main way to learn to say yes when someone offers to help.

You can do anything, but you cannot do everything.
—David Allen

That quote is spot on. If you focus, you can do anything. You can focus and get it done, but you can't do everything. You have to stop trying to be the hero and do it all yourself. There are others who can actually do a great job. I had to learn this through my journey with my dad. In fact, it was interesting because through the years, we had a lot of different caregivers come in and support us in caring for my dad. We all had different personalities, and to be blunt about it, some of them were not my favorite.

There were some who talked non-stop. With my personality, I don't deal well with that. I'm more of a deep talker. I don't want to have surface-level conversations, but it was fun to watch my dad respond to those people who constantly talked. He joined in and laughed; they were silly together. Those surface conversations brought a whole different mood to him.

Dad and I were more about getting things done or playing games. That in-between silliness is just not one of my strengths, so it was enjoyable to see the various personalities bring out different things in my dad. In truth, I wasn't always the best person to do some of the things my dad needed for his care.

But I was the best person to do certain things with him. When it came to getting him to follow directions or help break things down into small pieces so he could understand something that was confusing to him, I did really well. When it came to the fun and playful times, I did not do as well as some of his other caregivers. Yes, he and I had our fun, but my strengths were so different from many of those who were part of our caregiving team.

Learning to see that I didn't have to do it all because I wasn't the best one to do it all definitely helped me say yes to allow help in through the doors. Sometimes, there are family members who might live long-distance but who want to help. They aren't right there and able to do the hands-on things, but they can still help. So be open to receiving the help you can get.

I'm going to challenge you. If you're in a season of caring, look outside for help and find those who can do things for you.

Who can do things like paying the bills? Maybe the person who lives out of town can pay them, or they can make phone calls, investigating services or activities for your parent. Allow people to offer respite for you. Let them come in for short periods of time and spend time with your parent while you use that time to get away and get some rest. There are opportunities to say yes to others helping. Just look for them.

It's important for you to find a right-hand person, too. Mine was my sister, Robin. Who's your Robin, your Tonto, or your Ethel? Find that person whom you can trust to do the quick and easy things. This will take stress and the over abundance of tasks off your plate, tasks such as picking up the dry cleaning, prescriptions, or the groceries. There are lots of little things that, if we let them, people who love us are more than willing to do.

Be on the lookout for your "listening ear." This person will allow you to vent because you need to process your emotions and then feel refreshed and ready to step back into your role. Take the help that is offered. People will ask, "Anything I can do for you?" Sometimes, your mind just goes blank. "No, I'm good. It's okay. Don't worry about it." Don't be so quick to say no. When people ask, think about it. Let them help if they can and if you have a need they can fill.

It's a helpful activity to sit down and think about what people can help you with. Write a quick "stuff I am letting go of" list, things that people could do for you, so that when someone asks you, you can say, "Just a minute. Let me look at my list and let you know."

I have resources in the back of this book, including a place to make and keep your list, or you can keep it on your phone so it's easy to access.

Raking the leaves, going to stand in line at the DMV to get car tags, and picking up medications are all easy tasks, but they all take time. Sometimes, that is time you just don't have. There are so many little tasks that we know need to be done, but we never find the time to do them. And don't just think of things that need to be done at your parent's home; what things do you need done at your home that you aren't able to get to because of the additional needs of your parent? By keeping an ongoing list of things you can let someone else do, when a person asks how they can help, you can say, "Actually, yeah. I need someone to do *this, this,* or *this.* Could you do any of those things for me?"

Accepting help is not always an easy thing, but it is always a helpful thing. Allowing people to help blesses them, as well as blesses you. Being open to help is definitely something that I learned through the season, for sure.

Stop Neglecting You

When you let someone else help, you stop neglecting you. There are things you need or need to accomplish through this season.

Caring for you is a non-negotiable in this season.

It is something that has to be done. You're not going to make it all the way through to the end of the journey if you don't take care of yourself. We talked about not forgetting your health, but I'm even talking about simple things of self-care, like haircuts.

It's kind of funny. When you're caring for your parents, those are things they need help with. They need to go to the doctor. They need to get their hair cut. They need to have their eyes checked. Here's a huge tip: When you're making their appointment, make your appointment. If it can be at the same time, that's ideal. If not, you've got to schedule time to bring somebody else in to help with the care so you can go and take care of yourself.

Neglecting self-care is not going to benefit you. This season is going to end, and if you haven't cared for yourself through this season, the negative impact on you will have a snowball effect on your overall health. Making sure you have taken care of yourself is the most important thing you can do to live a happy, healthy life after the season is over.

Actually, self-care action items are great things to put on your *To Do* list. Having them on the list means they won't be forgotten. You can ask for help in all of these areas, as well, even if that means simply finding someone to keep you accountable. Ask them to give you a reminder, "Check with me, and make sure I've done these things." This is a great way to ensure you're not neglecting yourself in this season.

When this season is over, you're still going to be the person you've always been.

You will have changed a little during the process. But you can't ever forget, there's a new season ahead. Keep yourself in the forefront of your care. Remember your relationships, your physical and mental health, and the other things that need to be maintained during this season of caring.

Stay Inspired

In the middle of this season, it's important to stay inspired. Losing your inspiration is a fast track to depression and unrest. Make a list of things that you love; then you'll know what to pull from when you have a few minutes for yourself. Plug into what gives you joy, even if it doesn't look the same as what it used to look like.

Creativity was one of the things that always fueled me, so having projects where I could sit down and create for just a few minutes here and there always brought me joy. Whether it was crocheting a dishrag or stamping a card to send to a friend, staying inspired was something that really helped me.

Do something that makes you feel like you.

When you become a caregiver, you need to embrace the self-imposed label—*caregiver*. But don't let that label become your identity. In reality, there are many other things that make you who you are. Do not let those things fall by the wayside; fight to keep them a part of you.

Sometimes, doing something different, something you haven't done in a while or haven't done before, can be a huge benefit. It could be visiting a museum or trying a new sport; it could be going to the YMCA to try a new class. Those new activities can help inspire you to keep on growing and learning, keeping yourself balanced as a person.

In order to stay inspired, you must know the signs of burnout. Burnout is a real thing, and it will definitely happen to you in this season if you're not careful. Be aware of that and know the signs. VeryWell-Health's website states there are seven signs of burnout to look for:

- Number one—you feel increased irritation, frustration, or anger over small things.
- Number two—your gentle, unhurried approach to providing care is disappearing or it's gone.
- Number three—you raise your voice at your loved one more often lately. Later, you feel upset and guilty.
- Number four—you often skip aspects of your loved one's care that are important to their wellbeing because they're just too difficult to do.

- Number five—your own mental health is declining. Perhaps you're struggling with increased anxiety, depression, or insomnia.
- Number six—your own physical health is declining. You have increased blood pressure, are needing additional medications, or you've injured yourself trying to transfer or do something physical to help your parent.
- Number seven—your own family is experiencing dysfunction, and your care for your loved one is harming your family.

My advice is to plug back into things that inspire you and give you energy and hope to recharge. Just be aware that burnout is a possibility, and if you're finding yourself dipping your toe in the waters of burnout, recognize it early on, pull your feet out, and take some time to become inspired again.

Find Hope

Hope is hard to put your finger on sometimes, especially in a caring season that involves aging parents. Many times, you know how this season will end, and it's not a pleasant one. You're not going to find a cure for aging. You're not going to walk away from this with younger parents, and you're not going to experience a relationship with them like what you had when you were younger.

There is finality that's coming as you walk with them to the end, but there doesn't have to be hopelessness in it all. This is just the way life works. Everyone is going to age, and we will all reach the end of our lives, and that's okay. There can be joy, hope, and love in the midst of this journey.

Don't get so deep in the thick of trying to deal with everything that you forget the love you have for the person you are caring for. You have to reframe the definition of hope. In this case, hope is not in finding a cure. It's not getting the happily ever after you dream about, but it's actually understanding how to live life in the moment. It's the time you get to spend with each other. It's the memories you'll make, and it's being able to live your life afterwards with no regrets.

Through this season, you are going to experience different heartaches. Acknowledge them, but don't just stop at the heartache. Look past the heartache for the hope that can come in the end. For me, Jesus Christ, my Lord and Savior, is my source of hope.

Being able to evaluate the heartaches that came through my season of caring has actually helped me to find hope in the way the Lord has helped me grow through the experience. He's allowed me to exchange the heartache for hope and for other things that have come out of the season of caring for my dad.

I've put together a list of heartaches that I exchanged for the beauty of hope. I hope these can show you that you can do the same.

Hope after my mom's terminal disease or diagnosis
...building a closer relationship with my dad.

Hope after watching my dad give up his job
to stay home and care for my mom
...learning what sacrifice really looks like.

Hope while my dad cares for my mom for twelve years in their home
...watching true love lived out.

Hope after feeding, bathing, and caring
for my mom's physical needs when my dad would let me
*...developing the ability to see someone's needs
without her being able to verbalize them.*

Hope after burying my mom when I was only twenty-eight
...seeing my mom through the eyes of others at her funeral.

Hope for life, even when my dad was diagnosed
with Alzheimer's seven years after losing my mom
...I'm valued and important to God,
even when the unthinkable happens.

Hope as Dad's disease progressed to needing twenty-four-hour care
...experiencing my husband's love and sacrifice
shining through for my family and me.

Hope after we decided to keep Dad at home
...growing a beautiful friendship with my sister.

Hope while cleaning up urine, poop, and blood after accidents
...stepping into Dad's needs and putting aside
any discomfort of my own.

Hope after burying Dad twenty years after Mom
...realizing I loved him well, walked him all the way home,
and have no regrets.

Hope while grieving the journey
...a heart to serve others as they walk their parents home.

There is always hope.

CHAPTER 16

Next Step

T hank you so much for reading *No Regrets: Hope for Your Caregiving Journey.*

It has been an honor to share my personal and professional experiences of caregiving with you in *No Regrets.* Though this season was one of the most challenging I have experienced, it was also one of the most rewarding. My heart's desire is for you to walk your parent all the way home and then walk back into your life fully present and with no regrets. I am passionate about supporting you and your parent in this season of life. I would love to connect with you and see if I can support you personally.

Now, it's time to take the next step. Go to CaringQuiz.com for my caregiving personality quiz.

I also offer a free monthly support group. Gather with others who are in a season of caring to transparently share joys and struggles. Find understanding, support, and encouragement as you journey together in this season. Go to ASeasonofCaring.com, click on "services," and scroll down to "support group." It's quick and easy to sign up!

I look forward to hearing from you!

Rayna

Rayna@ASeasonOfCaring.com

P.S. If you enjoyed this book, I'd appreciate it greatly if you would write a review. Getting feedback from readers is amazing, and it also helps others pick up this book as they journey through their seasons of caring.

Reader Resources

Stuff I'm Letting Go Of

Task	Date	To Whom

Decision To Be Made

PROs	CONs

Core Values to Consider:

If you'd like to learn more about how to determine your core values, visit www.ASeasonofCaring.com/CoreValues and use coupon code Book to take the course for free.

Relationship Check-in

1. List those who are in this Caring Season with you.
2. Now rank 1 (being awful, I would rather not see them) to 10 (things have never been better).
3. Create a next step to reconnect or communicate with each person on the list.

Name	1-10	Next Step

Create Your Personal Manifesto

Use the space below to answer these questions and move you toward creating your own Personal Manifesto: List your top 5 core values. Jot down the roles that you play in life. What do you wish to be true of you? What is true of you? What do others say about you?

Now try turning the most important information from above into statements.

I am _____ _____ who _____ _____.

Find more detailed directions at:
https://overwhelmed.website/personal-manifestos/

If you want to learn more about how to determine your core values, visit www.ASeasonofCaring.com/CoreValues and use coupon code Book to take the course for free.

God's Simple Invitation to Find Peace with Him

God Loves you

Sin has separated us from God but not from His love.
Romans 3:23 KJV says, "For all have sinned, and come short of the glory of God," But, John 3:16 KJV tells us, "For God so loved the world, that He gave his only begotten Son, that whosoever believes in Him should not perish, but have everlasting life." Romans 6:23 NLT "For the wages of sin is death, but the free gift of God is eternal life in Christ Jesus our Lord."

Jesus provided the way

Since Jesus is God the Son who became human and lived a sinless life, He is the perfect and only sacrifice for our sin.
Romans 5:8 KJV says, "But God commended his love toward us, in that, while we were yet sinners, Christ died for us." When Jesus died on the cross, He made the payment in full for all sins, for all people. He then overcame death and rose on the third day.

By faith trust in Jesus

Romans 10:9 says, "If you declare with your mouth, 'Jesus is Lord,' and believe in your heart that God raised Him from the dead, you will be saved."

Now it is up to you

If you realize you have sinned and want to be restored to having a relationship with God and believe that Jesus is the sinless Son of God who died for your sins and rose again, you can trust in Jesus to save you from the penalty of sin. In Romans 10:13, God promises that He will bestow His grace on those who do so—"Everyone who calls on the name of the Lord shall be saved."

Seek to grow in knowledge and understanding

A relationship with God is like all relationships—it takes time and attention to grow. Matthew 11:28-29 says, "Come to me, all you who are weary and burdened, and I will give you rest. Take My yoke upon you and learn from Me, for I am gentle and humble in heart, and you will find rest for your souls."

You will learn best in community. Seek out a local church to grow in love with the Lord daily.

If you've accepted the above invitation and want to know how to move forward in your Christian faith, or if you would like to know more about a personal relationship with Jesus Christ, please email me at Rayna@ASeasonofCaring.com.

Things I Love To Do Or Bring Me Joy!

Recommended Reading

Being Mortal: Medicine and What Matters in the End by Atul Gawandea

The Forgotten Commandment by Dennis Rainey

Undone: A Story of Making Peace with an Unexpected Life by Michele Cushatt

The Best Yes: Making Wise Decisions in the Midst of Endless Demands by Lysa TerKeurst

Understanding Your Grief: Ten Essential Touchstones for Finding Hope and Healing Your Heart by Alan D. Wolfelt, PhD

Overwhelmed: How to Quiet the Chaos and Restore Your Sanity by Kathi Lipp and Cheri Gregory

The Caregiving Season: Finding Grace to Honor Your Aging Parents by Jane Daly

Caring for Our Aging Parents by Michele Howe

About the Author

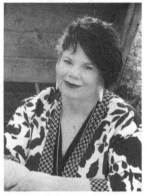

R ayna Neises is an author, certified coach, the host of "A Season of Caring" podcast, and speaker who is passionate about supporting daughters and sons in a season of caring with their aging parents. Rayna lost both of her parents to Alzheimer's disease twenty years apart. After her season of caring for her dad through his journey, she founded A Season of Caring Coaching where she offers encouragement, support, and resources aimed at preventing family caregivers from aimlessly wandering through this important season of life.

Rayna lives on a farm in southeast Kansas with her husband, Ron, and small pack of dogs. She is the baby of her family, but most would never guess that. She is a former teacher and enjoys crafts of all kinds and spending time with her grandkids most of all.

CPSIA information can be obtained
at www.ICGtesting.com
Printed in the USA
JSHW042249110521
14605JS00003B/106

9 781631 953446